Dying to Live

Georgia Comfort
with Philip Comfort

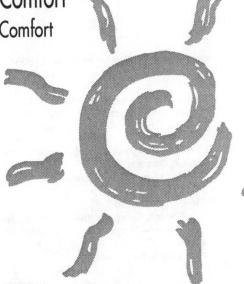

Tyndale House Publishers, Inc.
Wheaton, Illinois

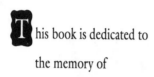his book is dedicated to

the memory of

Dr. Barbara Brown,

Brenda Stahr, and Ryan Moll

Library of Congress Cataloging-in-Publication Data
Comfort, Georgia, date
  Dying to live / Georgia Comfort with Philip Comfort.
     p. cm.
  ISBN 0-8423-0798-2
  1. Comfort, Georgia, date—Health. 2. Breast—Cancer—Patients—
United States—Biography.   I. Comfort, Philip Wesley. II. Title.
RC280.B8C62   1992
362.1'9699449'0092—dc20
[B]
                                                                    92-10140

Printed in the United States of America

98 97 96 95 94 93 92
9   8   7   6   5   4   3   2

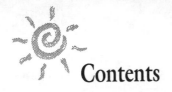

Contents

Foreword

This book tells the story of a woman who faced breast cancer and decided to "go for the cure." Her story is passionate, direct, and personal. It touches every one of us—whether we are patients, family members, friends, or medical caregivers—for all of us, at one time or another, must deal directly with someone who is facing a medical crisis and even death.

Be prepared to get involved with this story. And be prepared to get to know Georgia Comfort well, as I have known her since high school. You will see that she is a "good person" with an extremely positive attitude, a person who didn't deserve to have this "bad thing" happen. You will know her as a patient whose medical problems are severe, whose chances of living very long are extremely low, according to all the medical statistics. You will also learn of her spiritual story, her faith in the healing power of God.

This book speaks deeply to me, both as a person and as a medical professional. On the practical side, Georgia's story has helped me to see cancer and medical treatment from a patient's point of view. She shows us that patients need tender love and honest truth—a delicate balance. Medical caregivers bearing bad news need to maintain that balance. Without taking away patients' hope with messages of gloom and doom, doctors and nurses must inform them clearly and directly of both the "cannibals chasing close behind" (the dangers of their disease) and the "river of crocodiles ahead" (the risks of medical treatments), one of the many revealing metaphors of this artful book. Patients need to maintain a positive attitude. And in the depths of their crises, patients need medical professionals they can trust.

Reading Georgia's story has also helped me to reflect on some of the more philosophical questions of modern medicine—the seeming contradictions between science and religion, between evolution and creation, between philosophy and faith. When life-shaking crises occur, we become inescapably aware of how frail our bodies really are. During these times of trial, especially when facing death, the apparent disparities in perspective between faith and science are replaced with the realization that our human understanding of this world is terribly limited in relation to eternity. Since death is unexplainable in human terms, it outstrips our ability to explain the meaning of life through science or philosophy. Facing death forces us to look in faith to a reality beyond ourselves. While science articulates the incredible order within this world, God is the glorious source of that order. Science declares the depth of God's glory.

Healing also encompasses both the spiritual and scientific realms. When healing occurs through medical treatment, it is a gift of the Creator just as is life itself.

Georgia describes one of the medical tools used in her care as "a product of human genius through which God would dispense His grace." One of the miracles of all living things is the capacity to heal. God has unveiled to people knowledge of many aspects of His incredibly complex creation, but the amount known is far less than the unknown. All who are involved in the healing process need to see that medical science works together with the healing power of God. Every tool God has given us—including medical science, prayer, and the power of the Holy Spirit—should be fully used.

Reading about Georgia's experience and her positive attitude will inspire you and help you to prepare for the challenges in your life.

William J. Stewart, M.D.

Acknowledgments

I am thankful to the following people for helping to make this book what it is:

My husband, Philip, for encouraging me to write this book, for his writing and editing, and for his poems

Lissa Johnson, for her word coloring and craft of writing

Dr. William Stewart, for his insight, faith, medical knowledge, and friendship

Wendell Hawley, for his interest and help in getting this book published

Dan Elliott, for his work as my editor at Tyndale House

Introduction
The Beginning

The seed came from a living plant and now lies dor-
mant, in a deathlike state underground. But with the
warmth of spring it ruptures, and the shoots that break
forth suckle nutrients from water and earth to form a
new living thing. Grass. Vegetables. Flowers. A tree.

A caterpillar wraps itself in the vestiges of death.
Time passes. Emerging from the cocoon is a creature of
life whose wings bear it up to the sky.

The unborn infant stretches one last time. Within
hours, she will emerge from the darkness. The safe
home that harbored her pushes her out into a new
world.

A man carries a heavy beam of wood, its splinters
spiking His back and shoulders. He is posted to the
wood and dies. Hours and days later, He walks from
His burial most certainly alive.

Much in nature tells us the process of death does
not lead to death but to life. I never anticipated that I
would become another example of *Dying to Live*.

I don't suppose the idea of breast cancer would ever
have crossed my mind if it hadn't been that two of my
relatives had died from it. But since they had, the

thought pursued me from the deep recesses of my brain. It would come to me in the middle of teaching piano to one of my better students. It would come to me in the middle of the night when the breast pain would wake me from a sound sleep. I tried in vain to put the thoughts to rest.

My physician had ordered a mammogram in 1984, when I was thirty-four, since I was experiencing pain in my left breast and my family history indicated I should have the test. The negative results told the doctor we had nothing to worry about.

The intermittent pain continued in my left breast for another three years. The physician continually reassured me that the further tests I requested were unnecessary. She backed up her decision with three facts: breast cancer never caused pain, there was no palpable lump, and the mammogram had been negative. She didn't hesitate to remind me who had the degree in medicine and who had the degree in music. On occasion, she slipped in small remarks about my overreaction to the pain.

I'll never forget thinking, "If she's wrong, and I do have cancer, I'll be so mad."

With continuing pain, I went to another doctor a few months later. After rehashing my family's medical history as well as my own, I requested a mammogram. Without hesitation he responded, "Absolutely."

The mammogram returned with one word of caution: *Suspicious.* The report noted calcification in my left breast and suggested a repeat mammogram in three months to see if there was any change.

A week later, I awoke with a damp spot on my

nightgown. Looking down, I noticed pus coming from my nipple. I returned to the doctor, who then ordered an immediate biopsy.

I was born Georgia Ann Riser in 1951 in the midwestern state of Ohio, to loving parents, George and Joan. My father raised me with the principle of caring for others, regardless of who they are or what their background. Wanting to befriend and help those who needed love and nurturing was not only a philosophy of life but a characteristic as natural as breathing. As a result, I had many friends in high school, and my class voted me homecoming queen.

I carried this philosophy of love and caring into my marriage at age twenty. I cared enough to help support the family for several years while my husband, Philip, went through undergraduate and graduate school. After completing his studies, Philip found his niche in two jobs: as an editor at a publishing house and as a professor of New Testament studies at a nearby college.

With Philip supporting us, I focused my time and energy on loving and caring for my three boys, Jeremy, John, and Peter. I enjoyed nurturing them, playing with them, and being their mom until they were all in school. Yet I also looked forward to the day my youngest, Peter, would enter first grade. That would mark the beginning of time spent on *me*. Time for rest, time for me to enjoy activities I wanted to participate in but hadn't been able to because of other family priorities.

Like most people, I had plans for my life. Plans that included expanding my private piano studio.

Exploring my music and how I could use it to serve the Lord and my students. Going to graduate school. Taking dance classes. Tagging along on my sons' sports activities. And it was all right there, just within my reach.

"You Have Cancer"

My right hand moved gracefully and effortlessly over the piano keys. My left didn't respond as quickly. The breast biopsy had slowed it down just a little. It had gone well, though. Since I didn't have a lump, the surgeon made a four-inch incision and removed several sections of tissue. I went home the same day as the surgery.

Now, on Thursday evening, as I played my favorite Chopin nocturnes, the phone rang. Often I let the answering machine pick it up while I played or taught piano. But this time the ringing startled me. My heart started beating faster as I crossed the living room to the kitchen phone. Without any preliminaries, the surgeon dealt the felling blow. "You have cancer."

My breath left me, sucked from my lungs by his powerful words. I sat frozen in the chair, barely able to put the phone back on the hook. Although he hadn't said so, the doctor might as well have said, "You are dying." I couldn't believe it. How could I, at thirty-eight, die? My life was just getting together. It wasn't the right time to die. *This isn't fair!* It was time for me to be me, not time for me to die.

I didn't want to be a statistic. I wanted the doctor

to call me back and tell me he was wrong. I didn't want to be the one in ten American women who would be diagnosed with breast cancer that year. And I certainly did not want to be one of the 144,000 who would die.

My Second Surgery: A Mastectomy

I could only think that I had been cursed. I had cancer, breast cancer—a killer of women! First my aunt and cousin had died of it. *Now it's my turn,* I thought. Somehow I had to escape.

I felt the disease invading my entire life. I did not invite it. Nevertheless it swooped in, uninvited, unwanted, like alien soldiers infiltrating a country.

The surgeon recommended that I have my left breast removed immediately in a type of surgery known as a modified radical mastectomy (removal of the breast and armpit, while leaving the pectoral muscle on the chest).

I wanted to get a second opinion from a breast specialist to be certain some other type of surgery wouldn't be better, or to see if radiation might eliminate the cancer. But the surgeon reassured me that he was a breast specialist, and he insisted that I take care of it right away. He explained that there had been no lump because the cancer simply filled all the milk ducts. The whole breast was involved. I had no other options. Since I had been very neglected by my general practitioner when I had complained to her for a few years about the pains in my left breast, I decided to trust the surgeon and get this insidious enemy off my chest. Fear of death as a result of having cancer was my impetus to act imediately.

On Friday, I spent the whole day calling different

surgeons and specialists. Each one recommended the same procedure. Saturday and Sunday I wandered about the house in a tumultuous daze. Little prayers exploded in my brain. *Oh Lord, what do I do?* It seemed like I didn't have any choice in the matter. If I wanted to be aggressive with the cancer, I had to get it out of my body. I couldn't allow myself to care what I would look like afterward. All I knew was that I wanted this horrible disease out of my body so I could live. Finally, I made the decision. *I don't want this cancer in my breast. Get it off me!*

Little Girl Waiting

Foolishly, I allowed my surgery to be scheduled for Monday afternoon. This meant I had to sit around all morning waiting for the horrible amputation to take place. *I'm going to be deformed.* Each minute trudged by like a child trying to make his way through a deep snow drift. *When I wake up, I'm going to be horribly deformed.* The anesthesiologist had warned me not to eat or drink anything after midnight. Fear had quenched my appetite but not my thirst. *It's going to hurt worse than anything I've ever felt before.* Every so often I gazed longingly at the drinking fountain.

Philip sat with me, stroking my hair, holding my hand, looking very, very scared.

"Philip," I said in a very tiny voice, "I don't want to go."

His eyes held all the gentleness he had for me. "Oh, honey, I wish you didn't have to go either. I wish you didn't have to do this."

Somewhere inside, a little girl had escaped and taken over the grown-up Georgia. Her voice pleaded with the only person who she felt could help her. "I don't want to go. Philip, don't let me go!"

"You've got to go." Philip swallowed hard, holding back his emotions. "You just have to do this. I wish you didn't have to do this. But you have to."

At eleven-thirty the nurse came to prepare me for the surgery. At almost three o'clock, she returned with an orderly. She motioned with her head toward me, and told him matter-of-factly, "You can put this case on the cart."

I mustered all the dignity I could while dressed in a hospital gown and said, "I am not a case, I am a person. And my name is Georgia. That is not a cart, it is a bed. And I would like you to dignify me and these other people a little bit better than that."

The startled nurse said nothing as I climbed into the bed. The large arms of the orderly gripped the bed and began to push. The little girl stared at the doors as they rushed past. I couldn't help feeling that the big bad wolf was at the end of the hall.

A Unique Approach to Surgery

The final steel doors swung open to let me in, like the jaws of the wolf stretching wide to swallow me whole. I fought to keep my fear under control, to keep it from becoming frantic. I didn't want this. I didn't want to go under the anesthesia with the memory of the nurse telling the orderly to "put this case on the cart." I wanted to be loved by the medical people. I felt I deserved to be cared for—not treated coldly, like some specimen ready for examination under a microscope.

In an instant, I thought of a bizarre solution. I didn't care how it would sound. I only cared about changing the fear to a more positive feeling. As the medical personnel bustled about the operating room, I spoke up, my voice sounding hollow as it echoed off the bare walls. "Would all of you please put your hands all over my body from my head down to my legs? While I'm going to sleep, I want you to tell me that you love me."

As the anesthesiologist put the mask over my face, he asked me to count backward from one hundred to determine the effects of the anesthetic. As I did, I felt ten pairs of hands gently touching me on my calves, thighs, abdomen, shoulders, and head. Their voices mingled with the same message, "We love you, Georgia. We love you."

Slowly the fear slipped away, melting into warmth and security. No longer was I a cold, clinical, impersonal case on the cart. I understood the hands that rested on me were hands that would cut me, but they were hands that also cared for me.

I entered the unknown depths of sleep, feeling very loved and comforted. I felt like a little girl in Mommy's lap. Mommy and Daddy were holding my hands.

Coping with Pain and Deformity

I awoke feeling OK about the surgery. It seemed to have gone well. I didn't have any pain because I used a

PCA (patient-controlled anesthesia) machine to give myself small doses of morphine. And my nurses were great! For having such a devastating surgery, I was doing tolerably well. The morphine not only dulled the pain but also gave a sense of euphoria to my entire being. At this point I was very happy. Happy to have the surgery over and to be feeling good. When I spoke to relatives and friends on the phone, they were surprised that I was so happy. Furthermore, I received the good news that there was no sign of cancer in the lymph nodes under my arm.

When I came home from the hospital, things changed completely. Because I was no longer on the morphine, I began to feel the pain. I started physical therapy to regain the range of motion in my left arm and hand, but every movement jolted me with pain and fear. Mixed in with the therapy were many strong and confused emotions. I feared the disease would return and spread. When I looked at myself in the mirror, I saw a flat chest with a long scar going from my sternum to under my arm. I felt such sadness and grief. The very ugly scar increased my feelings of being assaulted and humiliated. What had I done to deserve this? How could I cope with life when I didn't feel like a whole person anymore?

Being an upbeat person, my outlook on life had always been positive. I tried to counter my sadness and sense of tragedy by telling myself, "OK, so you have only one breast now, but the other one wasn't big anyway. Don't be so upset about it." Or I would say, "At least they got all the cancer. So what if you only have one breast."

Because the doctors detected no other sign of cancer in my body, my fears about dying remained but didn't overwhelm me. I consoled myself with reminders that I was now labeled an "early-detection case."

At the end of March, about a month after surgery, our family took a vacation in Florida. I asked them if they would mind if I wore my two-piece bathing suit without a false breast. My sons and husband said no, they wouldn't feel embarrassed to be seen with a woman whose bathing suit wrapped flat against her left chest. Their support helped me accept my new, altered appearance. They helped me see that the real Georgia was the woman inside the body, and my deformity didn't change my relationship with them.

Philip made an effort to encourage me continually. He told me that no matter what happened, he still loved me and cared for me. Although I had been mutilated, although I had become deformed, he saw me and treated me like a complete woman. He wrote this poem after my mastectomy:

> you are loved
> not because your form's immortal
> like an ancient marble goddess,
> nor because you've lived in heaven
> where time is still and tears are gone;
> you are flesh and soul and spirit—
> flesh with hurts and soul with pains,
> yet your spirit, inspired and spirating,
> breathes a sweet refrain:
> you are life put to music
> you are song that others sing

7

you're what musicians dream of making—
a symphony in living being.
you have moved me with the beauty
of a life lived for Him
who once piped mystic music
to the blind and deaf and dumb.
I have heard and now I'm dancing
to the song you long have been.

Chapter

2

The Disease Spreads

Breast cancer typically spreads first to the lymph nodes under the armpit. Since my lymph nodes were "negative," we believed the surgery had removed all the cancer and that I was going to be fine. The surgeon had told us, "I think we got it all. I left only a vein and an artery underneath your arm."

However, the same week that I had my surgery, the *New England Journal of Medicine* published a study indicating that women who were node negative were advised to take additional cancer-killing medicines (adjuvant chemotherapy) to prevent the spread of the disease.

So a couple of weeks after my mastectomy, I went to see a nationally renowned medical oncologist (a doctor who specializes in cancer). I assumed this doctor would follow the treatment outlined in the *Journal of Medicine,* but she didn't. She explained that I had a 3 percent chance for a recurrence of cancer and that adjuvant chemotherapy could, at best, reduce that chance only by one percent.

Others were not so sure. Since my report showed the breast cancer had gone beyond the mammary ducts and had invaded my breast tissue, my mother, mother-in-law, and sister were disturbed that the oncologist did not advise me to get chemotherapy. I again accepted a trained physician's opinion over that of my family and my own intuition, and I did not have any chemotherapy.

Philip clung to the doctor's assessment that I was an early-detection case, anxious to put it all behind us. My sons were relieved that everything was going to be fine. The only one who struggled with uncertainty was me. For the sake of my family I tried to hide my anxiety and not let it take over—because cancer can become an all-consuming concern. Above all, I wanted to remain positive and life-giving to my family and others.

Two months after my surgery, I noticed something strange about my right breast around the nipple. It seemed to be changing color a little bit. One day it was reddish-brown; the next, yellowish-brown. Every day it seemed to be a different color. *CANCER* loomed like a theater marquee in my mind, so I returned to the surgeon who did my mastectomy and asked him what he thought this changing nipple might mean.

"Georgia, if it was anyone else, I would tell them not to worry about it," he said. He put his hand on his chin, rocked back on his heels, and continued, "But since you just had Paget's disease [a precancerous condition of the nipple and areola] on the left breast, I want to make sure you don't also have it in the right breast."

He left the examining room and went straight to his office to schedule me for a major biopsy of the right breast as soon as possible. I sat on the exam table and stared at the floor. My thoughts swirled with anxiety and fear. *This horrible disease might be spreading*. I went back to surgery for a biopsy similar to the one I had for the left breast.

At this same time, my husband's brother, Rich, was kind enough to send airline tickets for me to visit his family in Paris, France. I didn't want to miss this opportunity to go back to France, so my surgeon said I could have the biopsy and go to Europe with the stitches in. Then, as soon as I got back from Europe, he would check my stitches and give me the results of the biopsy. I readily agreed with his plan. I wanted to have a good time in France, so I didn't want to know the results before I left.

Philip and the boys graciously let me go to France by myself for those ten days. I had a wonderful time—thanks to such a wonderful family. Both Philip's family and mine have been very strong and supportive, as well as being very generous with their finances in assisting our family through some very difficult times.

After a refreshing vacation in France, I called the surgeon. Again, he dealt the blow without mincing words. "Georgia, you have Paget's disease on the right breast also. But I don't know if there is carcinoma inside the breast. I suggest you have a mastectomy of the right breast in the near future because carcinoma usually follows Paget's disease."

I couldn't breathe.

My Fourth Surgery: Another Mastectomy and Breast Reconstruction

This time I refused surgery before obtaining a second opinion. I eagerly drove an hour to see the medical oncologist I had seen after my first mastectomy. I again asked her for chemotherapy. While she again refused, she recommended I have the right breast removed in the near future. If not, there was a strong possibility the cancer would show up later in this breast. The oncologist arranged for me to see one of the surgeons at her hospital, a marvelous man who became my oncology surgeon and my primary, trusted medical ally.

I had been reading everything I could get my hands on and talking to everyone I could find about breast cancer. Somewhere during my massive information intake I learned that a woman could have breast reconstruction during the same surgery as the mastectomy. The reconstruction is done by putting in silicone implants under the pectoral muscle immediately following the mastectomy. After consultation with the plastic surgeon, the oncology surgeon, and the medical oncologist, I decided to have double breast reconstruction at the same time as my second mastectomy. At age thirty-eight I felt I was too young to be flat-chested for the rest of my life. I wanted my body to have some feminine curves.

This surgery left me in excruciating pain. I couldn't roll to the left; I couldn't roll to the right. I had to stay flat on my back in the hospital bed. Adding to my misery was a faulty PCA machine. No morphine was being administered for six hours. Finally the medical staff requested another one for me, and that one also was not working properly. My mother, Philip, and my son Jeremy took turns shoving their hands under my back to try to diminish the crescendo of pain. It was a living hell to come out of bilateral chest-wall surgery without pain relief. My family left that evening reassured by the nurse that the third machine was operating fine and that I would be kept as comfortable as possible.

I woke up shortly after midnight, alone in my room with my guard rail down. The nurse call button was on the rail below my reach, so I couldn't get to it. My sheets were wet with sweat. I was shivering and writhing in pain, but not able to turn to the left or to the right. I called out in my weakened voice, but the exertion made me dizzy. It was a waking nightmare.

At last the nurse came in. I asked for pain relief and for clean sheets. She explained that there was a power shortage that night and that's why the morphine wasn't being administered. She said she could help me with the pain, but that to change sheets was not her job. I would have to wait for the seven o'clock shift to come on duty before I could get off of my wet sheets! I was cold, in excruciating pain, and now angry as well. By morning I was crying hysterically. Rather than fixing the problems that had caused my nightmare, a psych nurse was called in to find out why I had been unable to handle the previous night. I vowed to myself that I would never enter another hospital—especially that one.

I had to start a physical therapy program again to regain movement in my arms. Both the left and right implants needed to be worked on to make them take the proper shape. And I had to work with my left and right arms to regain my flexibility and break up the scar tissue. I was very diligent with this therapy, even extra-diligent because I wanted to get back to teaching piano. I worked hard to regain mobility in my arms and hands so that I could adequately demonstrate piano skills to my students and play the piano for my own enjoyment. I wanted desperately to return to some sense of normalcy. I wanted to be whole again—body, soul, and spirit.

Chapter

3

The Disease
Spreads Even Further

By September of 1989, two months after my bilateral reconstruction surgery, I felt fit enough to work at the high school where I taught piano and accompanied the choirs. I also reopened my private piano studio. It was good to be back at work again and to feel like a normal human being.

Only three weeks after I started teaching school, I was hit with more bad news. During a routine visit to my medical oncologist, her fingers danced along my neck and collarbone. Then they stopped, reversed, and began to probe. "Georgia," she asked, "how long have you had this lump in your neck?"

Shaken, I replied, "I didn't know I had a lump in my neck."

"Well, it's right here along your collarbone," the doctor responded.

The day before, I had cut my finger on a knife while rushing around trying to get breakfast ready and everybody out the door for school and work. We surmised that I might have a little infection that had swollen the lymph nodes. Although I knew this was a silly idea, the thought of facing cancer again scared me

15

greatly. I wanted to think of any other reason that could cause the nodes to swell.

The doctor interrupted my thoughts. "You need to see the surgeon tomorrow morning. Let him take it from here because I will be out of town for a while."

The next day, concern filled the doctor's comments. "Georgia, from the way it feels I do believe it is a recurrence of cancer. The only way I can tell for sure is to go in, excise the nodes, and have them biopsied. Then we'll know for sure." Only ten days earlier this surgeon had checked me and had not reported anything, so he thought that the lumps must have suddenly appeared. The rapid growth of the tumor meant that it was aggressive and malicious and that it had *not* been caught in time.

Seeking Jesus in Desperation

This bad news stripped both my husband and me of the hope we had been living with. Philip became desperate; he didn't want me to die. He wanted to find Jesus—to contact Him and have Him come and heal me. For several days he prayed in desperation, "Jesus, if You were here on earth, as You were in Galilee two thousand years ago, I would get You and bring You to my wife—or I would bring my wife to You. I know that if You laid Your hands on her she would be healed. But You are not here like that now—in the flesh. So how do I find You? Because I know that one touch from You would heal her."

He prayed this over and over. As he prayed, he became convinced that he had to find someone who had the gift of healing—someone who knew Jesus as the Healer.

One night, as we were lying in bed, he told me how desperate he felt. I said, "Philip, I really feel that between you and Jesus I'm going to be healed. I don't think you need to go find a healer because, with the power of Jesus in my life and the power of Jesus in you, I believe that I will find my healing. Philip, I will depend on you and the Lord to heal me."

Philip didn't deliberate. He said, "Well, OK. I'll pray for you." He put one hand on my neck on the spot that was presumed to have malignant lymph nodes, and he lifted his other hand toward heaven.

As I lay there with my eyes closed, I felt ready to be the receiver. I believed with full faith that Philip would contact the Lord. Philip started to pray. I don't remember the exact words of his prayer. But before we knew it a strong surge—almost like an electrical current—flowed from Philip into me, continuing for several minutes. We both sensed within the room peace, authority, and an overwhelming, awesome Presence. We knew it was the Presence of the Lord. It was as if Jesus Himself entered into our room, leaving His throne in heaven to come make a personal visit to us.

All of a sudden, the desperation and anxiety that had consumed us disappeared. In their place glowed a warm peace. We no longer struggled. We felt calm.

"Philip, I think Jesus was here," I whispered.

Philip whispered back, "He's still here."

So I thought I had better be quiet. As I lay there, bathing in the current of strength and power of the Presence, I thought of God's glory. I didn't see any glory, but I sensed the fullness of a very strong, glorious Person. Then, as the Presence slowly faded away, we became aware once again of our surroundings. We both rejoiced that we had experienced a visitation—a strong, intimate, personal visitation from the Lord. We lifted our hands up and praised the Lord. We wanted to give Him glory and honor and thanks for showing Himself to us in that way.

Because of this event, Philip believed that I had been healed, but I didn't have the same belief. I had spent too many hours contemplating the possibility of recurrence and the debilitating effects this disease could bring into my life to believe healing would come that simply. I was grateful for the experience but didn't necessarily equate it with a full healing. Rather, I took it as a wonderful faith-refreshing experience. I knew without a doubt that I believed solidly and totally in the resurrection of Christ and in the resurrected Christ Himself. And I knew that wherever I was going to go, He would lead me there and be there with me. If I had to die, I was not afraid because I would be with Jesus. And if I lived, it would be because He decided to heal me. I had found extraordinary peace.

Philip was happy, praising the Lord and saying I was healed. I was happy and praising the Lord, but I was not saying that I was healed. I chose to have the surgery.

My Fifth Surgery

I decided not to have general anesthesia for this surgery. The surgeon assured me that it would be simple and easily done with a local pain killer. Besides, after four surgeries in six months, each requiring anesthesia, I felt it would be better for my body to do without. It didn't take long to regret that decision because the surgery turned out to be extensive. The surgeon chose to excise a few nodes that were nestled deep in my neck. He kept giving me shots of Novocain throughout the surgery as the simple procedure stretched into a more complicated one. Happily, my surgeon is a very funny man. He humored me throughout the surgery by cajoling me and telling me funny stories.

That surgery deepened my respect for this surgeon—not only because this was the second surgery he had done on me in a two-month period, proving himself to be an expert surgeon, but also because he was a humorous and compassionate human being. He cared about me as a person, not just a case on a cart. I became attached to this doctor and requested that he be my primary physician. In the event that there would be more problems from my disease, I needed somebody I could trust for my treatment. He was the first physician to earn my complete trust.

After the surgery, Philip and I anxiously waited in the recovery room for the doctor to come and give us the report about the lymph nodes he had removed. Philip hoped for a miracle; I expected to hear the truth.

The doctor walked in, his long strides quickly covering the distance between beds. Without hesitation, he took me by the hand and said, "I'm very sorry to tell you that it is a recurrence of cancer."

I blinked several times, trying to get enough courage to ask the ultimate question but unsure if I wanted the answer. "Does that mean I am going to die soon?"

Without letting go of my hand, he gently replied, "No, that's not the nature of the disease. But it does mean that your prognosis has changed very much. There are a few women who have survived long-term after having a regional recurrence of breast cancer. Let's hope for the best. Don't despair. You should have some tests and scans done in the near future to see if there is cancer anywhere else. Hopefully there isn't. And then we'll schedule an appointment with your medical oncologist to see what kind of treatment you should receive."

The doctor squeezed my hand, shook Philip's, then left. He had told us not to despair, but we couldn't help it. The report told us the cancer had spread to my neck and saturated two lymph nodes, causing them to become enlarged and grow together. It was obvious the cancer had been there for quite a while but had gone unnoticed. I could only wonder, *Why didn't my doctors find this earlier? Where will the cancer show up next?*

Philip, having expected a miracle and not seeing one, was despondent. He told me later that his confidence had never been so shaken. However, his faith was somewhat restored later that week when the test results came back indicating that there was no sign of cancer anywhere else in my body. The CAT scans of the lungs and liver and the bone scan were all negative. Thus we believed that the cancer in the lymph nodes was the sign of only a regional spreading, or metastasis. Philip wanted to believe that all the cancer was now gone. I still had doubts because I know breast cancer is a systemic disease—it travels to the bone, brain, liver, and lungs—and it kills. Knowing that cancer could be spreading in my body was very frightening because I never forgot that there is no cure for cancer.

Cold Waves of Raw Fear

Shortly after the surgery, Philip and I decided to take a weekend away by ourselves so that we could have the freedom to cry and express our feelings of despair together. We didn't want the children to be exposed to our raw, confused, and terrified emotions.

We went to a nearby resort town. Not knowing what to do, it seemed all we did that weekend was cry, eat, and stare at each other. We didn't know the proper protocol for relating to one another with Death eavesdropping on our conversations.

We couldn't do anything except sit there and experience the cold waves of raw fear billowing over us. Philip held me as I trembled with the cold of my emotions. I had never felt so horrible. We were both frightened and debilitated. We were so devastated we could hardly function.

We worried about what was going to happen, and we wondered how much more we could tolerate. We were exhausted from the past six months of dealing with the disease. How could we continue to raise our three boys and treat my illness at the same time? We reminded each other of the spiritual visitation we had, and we prayed and tried to regain the peace of Christ.

I'm so grateful that throughout the most tumultuous times of dealing with cancer, we were able to find a sense of peace. Sometimes it would take an hour . . . two days . . . maybe even a few days, but ultimately we could come in contact with the peace that is found only in Christ.

4

My Three Sons

Knowing that cancer was in my system, I wanted chemotherapy. My oncologist was back in town, and I quickly made an appointment.

The oncologist stared down at my file, then looked up at me, her face filled with knowledge I did not want to know. "Georgia, we thought you were an early-detection case. You're not."

I sat frozen to the chair. I watched her every move yet was unable to respond to anything she said.

"I don't think we can buy you any more time."

I asked, "Don't you know anyone who had breast cancer in their neck nodes and survived?"

She stared at the floor and answered grimly, "A few."

I appreciated her honesty. I hated the truth.

Back at home, I was hardly aware of the evening as it passed. I went to bed, hoping the nightmare would disappear while I slept. Instead, it filtered into my subconscious and created a heart-wrenching dream. In my dream, my doctors told me I would die very soon. They encouraged me to send my children away so they wouldn't see me suffer. So I arranged for them to take a bus to go to their usual summer camp in a nearby state. They were all very excited to go and had no idea they would never see me again. I watched them wave good-bye, knowing that was the last time I would see them. That knowledge absolutely shattered me. It tore my heart in pieces!

I woke up shaking; it was the worst dream I'd had in my whole life. I rolled over and shook Philip, told him my dream, and urged him to pray for God to spare my life. Philip slipped out from under the covers and began to pray. His prayers continued until just before dawn.

After that dream, I began almost unconsciously to distance myself emotionally from my three sons and even from my husband. At the time I didn't understand what I was doing, but later I realized I was trying to protect them and myself from the possibility of having to leave one another. My sons were dependent on me in many ways. The thought of them not having me as their mother overwhelmed me. The pain was so great that I shut down emotionally, especially toward the boys. I felt Philip could handle my possible death better than the boys, so I did not withdraw as much from him.

This emotional withdrawal continued for quite a while as I went in and out of the hospital. When I came back after treatments or surgery, I felt drained. I needed to protect myself, and I hoarded what little energy I had for myself. On days when I had more energy, I was able to pay attention to my family, and then beyond them to my piano students and my friends.

Although I was home, I would stay in my room resting for many hours, trying to recover from what-ever treatment I had been given. As a result of my debil-itated condition, the children suffered. They feared losing their mother, and they suffered also the rejection associated with my absence.

The boys internalized much of their pain. Because of their love for me, they were careful not to verbalize their frustration about having a nonfunctional mother. Knowing I had been through so much, they wanted to protect me from further agitation. Because they didn't want me to share their pain as well as bear my own, they kept it from me. It wasn't until much later that I realized they had been through an ordeal of their own.

Jeremy

My oldest son, Jeremy, was sixteen years old at the time. Tall and athletic, he would sometimes cry after football practice. I am grateful that his coach was a very understanding man. When Jeremy would break down and start crying due to my absence and his fear of what was going to happen to me, his coach related stories of his personal experience with testicular cancer. He shared how treatment took care of the disease, and that he was now doing well. This close relationship with someone who had fought cancer and won gave Jeremy hope for his mother, and it also gave him a strong adult who could sympathize with him.

The members of Jeremy's hockey team understood when Jeremy would suddenly get tears in his eyes, or when he just needed to talk about his fears related to his mother's illness and possible death. His closest friends, Greg and J.J., supported Jeremy and allowed him to open his heart to them.

Jeremy also turned to music to help him cope,

especially two songs composed by Michael Bolton. For a few months, every day after school he would sing along with these songs to help relieve his anxiety and sadness. The first song was "How Am I Supposed to Live without You?" As he sang along, he cried, thinking about my possible death and what life would be like without having a mother who dearly loves him and whom he dearly loves in return.

In the next song, "When I'm Back on My Feet Again," he would slightly change the words and imagine the person in the song to be me. He moved from the first song, which verbalized his fears, to the second song, which helped him visualize me recovering from my disease.

John

My second son, John, was eleven at the time. John is my perfectionist. He is a straight-A student and an excellent athlete. He dealt with his frustrations by trying to be better—the best in school and the best in sports. Yet there were many times when he would experience strong, sullen moods and obvious depression. Then we knew that everything was too much for him to bear. Intermittently, Philip and I would take time to sit down and talk to John about my disease and give him a chance to vent his feelings and frustrations about having a mother who didn't meet his needs.

John is a very sensitive person who deeply felt my pain along with his own. One evening we spent some precious time together, holding and loving each other as we wet our hair with each other's tears.

Peter

My youngest son, Peter, was six going on seven when I was diagnosed. We had been very, very close. I was his special mommy, and he was my special little boy. I had a close relationship with the other boys, as well, but since Peter was still so young, the closeness seemed more obvious at the time. Peter was too young to really understand the seriousness of my illness; it was my absences that disturbed him. Many times he would say, "Mommy, are you going to be a normal mommy again? Mommy, are you going to come to my school? When are you going to be like a real mom again?" Often he wanted to sleep with me to make up for the days I had been away at the hospital or away from the house to recuperate.

As time went on, Peter seemed to be more and more frustrated, which he expressed in aggressive behavior and manic energy. People who didn't understand what we were going through couldn't understand Peter's behavior.

Peter appreciated any kind of attention I could give him. Whenever I came to his school for one of his recitals or shows or visited his classroom to express parental interest, he'd grin from ear to ear. He was so happy when I displayed any signs of being a normal mom—a mom who participated in the life of her child.

I was always an active fan of my sons' athletic endeavors—whether hockey, football, or soccer. But for two years I rarely showed up at any of their sporting events. They tried their best to be big about it and understand, but deep inside they took it as a form of rejection. Why would I choose to stay home and take care of myself rather than go out and watch them do their sports? They saw the other mothers there, cheering and showing support, bringing the Kool-Aid, and being Team Moms. Why couldn't their mother be there too?

The ambiguity of the whole situation created a lot of anxiety for my sons. They eventually began making comments here and there that let me know how frustrated they were. But for the most part they kept their feelings inside. My sons loved and cared for me so much that they tried to hide their pain. They shed silent tears and whispered silent prayers. This silence showed they understood and cared, for if they had told me how they really felt, I would have agonized more than I was already.

I don't know if there is a stronger love than that of a mother for her children. This love has broken my heart many times over during the past few years, because of the times I have had to be away and because of considering the possibility of separation by my early death. But this love has also inspired me to fight for my life—to live for my three beautiful, wonderful children. I desperately wanted to stay here on earth with them. I was ready to do anything to lengthen my days. I visualized being at Jeremy's wedding, John's college graduation, and Peter's high-school graduation. I so desperately wanted to continue being their mother on a day-to-day basis, and I wanted to be there at the celebrated moments of their lives.

5

My Friend Barb

Sometimes a friendship is created that surpasses all other friendships. It is an intertwining of lives, like the climbing limbs of wisteria. It is a connection so intimate that being together produces fragrant blossoms that would have been impossible before the friendship. A proverb from the Bible confirms this unique relationship: "There is a friend who sticks closer than a brother" (Proverbs 18:24). My special friend was Barbara.

We started our friendship on a professional basis. Barb was my family's dentist and my son's orthodontist. I taught piano to Barb and her daughter, Colleen. Seeing each other so often helped the friendship deepen.

Eighteen months before my cancer diagnosis, Barbara entered the hospital to await the birth of her second child. The physicians, anticipating complications with a high-risk delivery, wanted Barb close by when the time came. While she waited for the birth, she discovered a lump in her breast. A biopsy confirmed the dreaded diagnosis: breast cancer. Yet before the doctors could treat the cancer, they had to deliver the baby, which they did by Caesarean section.

Six days later, Barbara had a modified radical mastectomy. I couldn't imagine recovering from a C-section and a mastectomy, and at the same time caring for a new baby. Barbara suffered, but she demonstrated incredible strength and recovered.

Barb Finds Christ

The night before her mastectomy she called me, hardly able to utter any words through her tears. As I listened to her fears, I knew what she ultimately wanted and needed, whether or not she realized it. She needed to know the Lord. In the past I had told her about having a relationship with Christ, but she would always say, "Georgia, that's nice for you that you believe in Christ and have a relationship with Him, but it's not for me."

Now she wanted to have the peace that I had in my life by knowing Jesus. "Well, Barbara, do you want to accept the Lord?" I asked.

She agreed to pray.

I offered to go ahead and pray, letting her repeat my words. I prayed a simple prayer: "Jesus, You are my Lord and Savior. I accept You into my life."

Perhaps Barbara had at some time in her days as a Catholic received the Lord, but what she needed now was the reality of Christ's presence in her life. Later, she told me that she prayed silently while I was praying and then experienced perfect peace. All her anxiety disappeared.

Bosomless Buddies

A year and a half later it was my turn. It "blew our minds" that two very close friends had breast cancer; the situation seemed quite unusual. When I had my first mastectomy, Barbara came to the hospital to visit me. Since we had fun joking around together, I said, "Barbara, do you remember when we were bosom buddies? Now we're bosomless buddies." We both laughed at the awful truth.

Our friendship deepened following my diagnosis, and our intimacy grew. We spent many hours talking about life and death, Christ and the Bible. We shared our viewpoints and ideas, our hopes and fears. We talked about eternal life and what it would be like after we die. We talked about what it would be like to go to heaven and to see the Lord.

Sharing Each Other's Sorrows

After one year of seeming remission, Barb's cancer spread rapidly. It soon invaded her mastectomy scar, lungs, eye, and liver. Chemotherapy at this stage wasn't strong enough to combat the advancing disease. She decided to undergo a bone-marrow transplant in an attempt to halt the disease. (This radical treatment is explained in chapter 7.)

I received word that my cancer had spread to the lymph nodes in my neck while Barb was in the hospital undergoing the bone-marrow transplant. I had promised Barbara that I was going to stop by and see her that afternoon. When I got there, she was receiving blood platelets. She was too debilitated to have company, so I didn't stay. I left a message with the nurse to tell her that I had been there and would come back.

The next day when I called her to see how she was doing, she asked me, "Georgia, I know you had an appointment. What did they say?"

"Oh, it's going to be OK," I said, hedging.

She intuitively knew I wasn't telling her the truth, that I was holding back.

I hesitated another moment, then felt I had to tell her the truth. "Well, Barb, they found a lump in my neck."

She started crying, "This isn't fair. This isn't fair for me, and this isn't fair for you!"

I tried to comfort her by telling her she was my example. "If I have to take more treatment, or whatever I have to go through, I feel I can make it because I've watched you go through this in such a brave way." I let her know that observing how she fought the disease motivated me to keep trying.

That night Barb's sobs haunted me. Because of the depth and honesty of our friendship, I couldn't lie to her. But I felt guilty that I had told her the truth, knowing how much the transplant had weakened her. I kept thinking, *Oh, I wish I hadn't told her. I wish I had kept the truth from her.* So that night I stayed up late and prayed that she would not be overwhelmed with sadness but that she would have the strength to get through the transplant.

It seems that the more friends suffer together, the closer they become. On one hand, it was terrible that my disease was spreading; on the other hand, it helped me relate to Barbara even more intimately. Our joint experience caused us to grow closer, and we each understood more keenly and painfully what the other person was going through.

6

Struggling with Mortality

When the doctors told me that radiation needed to be administered to my left neck and chest area, I consented. I only needed to hear they felt the cancer was spreading. They explained that the way a cancer spreads can tell them much about the progress of the disease. In my case, not having cancer in the axilla lymph nodes after the primary surgery, then discovering cancerous nodes in the neck, told them that not all of the cancer cells from the original site had been removed.

At first the radiation treatment didn't seem to affect me, but as each week went by I noticed I felt more tired. Soon my skin began to redden and burn, especially on my neck and underneath my breast and armpit. It felt and looked like the worst sunburn I ever had—only this sunburn didn't go away. I had to be careful to apply a cooling gel, and I had to choose clothes that wouldn't rub the burned areas.

One day, while waiting for my turn to go in for treatment, I sat in the brown vinyl chair crying silent tears. The supervising doctor—who was not the radiation oncologist treating me—came by and said, "Young lady, why are you crying?"

I wiped away a tear and looked up into his face. Expecting a compassionate listener, I replied, "Well, I have three sons, and I was told there isn't much hope for me now. I'm just devastated."

Half-jokingly he said, "Well, don't worry. I don't think you're going to die from cancer because the doses of radiation we are giving you will kill you first."

I stared at him in disbelief. How could he be so cold and cruel? His comment dragged insensitivity to new depths.

A couple of days later he came by again. Without expression, and without my asking for his opinion, he told me, "I did some research for you. As it stands right now—with the cancer going to the lymph nodes in your neck and probably spreading elsewhere through your system—you have about a 20 percent chance of survival."

That was really terrible to hear! I didn't know if he wanted to give me more bad news or if he was trying to be sincere and make up for what he had said two days before. I had not asked any of my doctors for my prognosis because I didn't want to know—and out of nowhere this doctor was giving me this prognosis! I didn't appreciate it, to say the least. I had experienced many negative emotions and had fought so hard for my spirit to remain positive against the constant fear and anger. For him to come along and give me such a terrible prognosis made this battle much more difficult. I had to fight all the harder to try to keep my spirit up.

Somehow I mustered up enough strength to get through the six weeks of radiation treatments. About the time I finished, Barbara came home from the bone-marrow transplant unit, knowing the transplant had failed. We both knew this meant her disease was terminal. I tried my best to support her and care for her, yet I was overwhelmed by the knowedge that my best friend was dying. I had never had any training on what to do for a dying friend. We tried to get together or talk on the phone as much as we could, but even that was incredibly difficult. Each time I saw her, spoke to her, or thought of her, I was reminded that she was dying from the same disease I had. I saw a future vision of myself, and I didn't want to think about it.

A Vacation in Hawaii

The intensity of my radiation treatments, coupled with the stress of suffering with Barbara, made me ready for some kind of a break. And then it came. For Christmas my sister's ex-husband, Mark, gave us a trip to Kauai in the Hawaiian Islands. My father graciously paid the bill for our condominium overlooking the sea. It was wonderful, and we felt so fortunate to have such a beautiful vacation provided by relatives. Yet because of my condition I could not fully enjoy the beauty of Kauai. I still suffered from extreme exhaustion caused by the radiation treatments, and I had picked up several infections as a result of my low resistance.

While there, I continued to struggle with thoughts of Barbara dying. And I struggled with thoughts of my own death. I felt aggravated and full of despair. And I questioned everything—especially the sad things and the sore things and the sick things of human life.

A lot changed for me one day when we had the

opportunity to take a guided helicopter tour of the lush island. The helicopter pilot skillfully dipped the craft into the craters of old rocky volcanoes, flew along emerald cliffs, and skimmed along the magnificent coast, where the cobalt blue ocean meets the towering mountains while waves crash on the shore. Words are not adequate to describe such extraordinary beauty, comprised of brilliant colors I had never seen.

As we flew along, I felt overcome by the power, majesty, and longevity of the earth. How different from the frailty, ugliness, and shortness of human life! How tiny and insignificant is the human body compared to the vastness of the earth and the universe. I had always considered my life to be so important and so worthy. While I was in the helicopter looking down at the earth and out over the glistening sea, I sensed just how small I really am.

All my struggles and perplexing questions about sickness and death seemed to dissipate as I spoke to the Lord. "God, it's OK," I whispered softly. "You are the Lord. You are God. You are the Creator—You made all of this! You are the Potter, and we are the clay. You gave us life, and You have the power to take our life."

At that moment, with all the beauty and majesty stretched out before me, I knew there had to be a purpose greater than my individual life. Although I was only a mere mortal, as tiny as a grain of sand in the universe, I knew it was a treasure to be a human being. To be human, even if there is suffering, is an incredibly valuable experience, and I was not ready for it to end.

By the time our vacation was over, I had a new plan for life. That day in the helicopter, I became a fighter. God's revelation of Himself through His creation inspired me to fight for my life. I did not want to leave this wonderful earth and God's wonderful plan for life on earth. I did not want to give up my life before it was time. And I would be willing to do anything to survive.

My Own High-School Reunion

When Philip and I got back from Hawaii, I had a couple of weeks to try to normalize. I had been sick there, and I was still sick when I came home. My goal was to get my household back together and get rid of the infections that I had. Then, near the end of January, I went to visit my parents in Cleveland, wanting to enjoy a normal time with Mom and Dad.

One evening, a couple of friends from my high-school years had planned to come to my folks' house to see me. They were eager to share with me news about our twenty-year class reunion, held three months before. I had missed the reunion while I was taking daily radiation. But before my friends arrived, flowers were delivered. Not long after that, a caterer delivered trays of deli foods, drinks, and desserts. I stared at all the food, wondering who had sent it and why so much.

Over the next couple of hours, I had my answer. The doorbell rang again and again. Groups of two and three people arrived, bearing hugs, kisses, tears, and funny remarks. By the time the evening was over, sixty-five of my former classmates had dropped in for an informal class reunion—all for me!

They explained to me that at the reunion word

had gotten around that the 1969 homecoming queen was suffering from breast cancer and was fighting for her life. The love my friends had for me in 1969 continued twenty years later, and they showed it by starting the Georgia Riser Comfort Cancer Fund, initiated and organized by my former classmate Jeff.

As we gathered in the dining room, one of my friends, Benny, read a letter from Jeff, who wasn't able to attend that evening. Jeff's words expressed his memories of me as a high-school student. He reminisced about the teenager who touched the hearts of those around her and who cared for people in all walks of life, wanting to help them, care for them, and be their friend. The letter brought tears to my eyes and to the eyes of many others in the room. I hung my head, afraid to look at the people who gathered to thank me for my friendship. An intensity of friendship and devotion filled the room, touching my heart and lifting my spirits. I felt unworthy of such love, but I was so grateful for it.

After the last of the friends left, my parents and I sat for a while, talking quietly. For all of us, it was a wonderful, warm, and strengthening experience. Knowing we had many people behind us gave us the fortifying sense that we were not alone in this fight.

Chapter

7

A Bleak Prognosis

I returned from Cleveland with all the experiences of
the past month giving me a solid, positive foundation
with which to face my disease. The first step included
tests to determine if the cancer had spread elsewhere in
my body. I wasn't prepared for the results. The bone
scan declared the disease had progressed to my sternal-
clavicular joint. When my surgeon told me this very
bad news, I knew my prognosis was worse than we had
previously thought. Now that the cancer had invaded
my bones, I might live only a year or two—for that is
all one can expect from conventional chemotherapy.
And I would probably die a slow, painful death.

The Bible Speaks

As I read my Bible, I discovered similarities between
my situation and one recorded in the Old Testament
book of 2 Kings, chapter 20—a story about Hezekiah,
the king of Israel.

Hezekiah trusted and obeyed the Lord. In fact,
none of the kings before or after him were as close to
God as he was. Hezekiah enjoyed a good life with

God's blessings until the age of thirty-four, when he became deathly sick. At that time, God sent the prophet Isaiah to speak to him.

Isaiah told the king, "Set your affairs in order and prepare to die. The Lord says you won't recover."

Turning his face to the wall, Hezekiah pleaded, "O Lord, remember how I've always tried to obey You and please You in everything I do." Then he broke down and cried.

Before Isaiah left the king's courtyard, the Lord spoke to him again. "Go back to Hezekiah, the leader of my people, and tell him that the Lord . . . has heard his prayer and seen his tears. I will heal him and . . . add fifteen years to his life."

Then the Lord directed Isaiah to prepare a poultice of figs and apply it to Hezekiah's boil. Isaiah did so, and Hezekiah was healed.

I saw the story as parallel to my own. When I found out that the cancer had gone to my bone, I asked the Lord to give me ten more years to live. I wanted ten more years—from 1990 to 2000—because in 2000 my youngest child would graduate from high school. I wanted to be a supporting part of his life until that day.

Furthermore, I believed that God could heal me through medicine. Since I had not received a direct healing from the Lord apart from medicine, I believed the Lord was leading me to receive divine intervention through medical application—the same way Hezekiah received his healing.

The Critical Decision

In all that I had learned about breast cancer, I learned that there are many choices of therapy ranging from very aggressive to very conservative. Above all, I wanted to live. All the decisions I had made combined to form one question I had to answer—and soon: *Am I willing to pay an outrageous price in order to live?* The outrageous price would entail very aggressive treatments through which, in a sense, the doctors would bring me to the brink of death in hope that my life would be restored. That trip to the brink of death would include incredible physical pain, sickness, and isolation. Worse, the doctors do not always know exactly where the edge is. In the course of some procedures, some patients are pushed too far by the treatment. But the patient is never an unwilling victim. She must choose whether or not she is willing to risk dying in order to live. The very aggressive procedure offered to me is known as a bone-marrow transplant.

The procedure was not new to me. Even before receiving the bad news about the cancer appearing in my bone, I had heard of the feasibility of bone-marrow transplantion. I also had learned quite a bit about it from Barb's experience. One oncologist had told me, "You are young and basically healthy. If you are brave, you should do a bone-marrow transplant. It could add ten to fifteen years to your life."

Now the time had come for me to make a firm decision about a bone-marrow transplant. I made an appointment with the bone-marrow transplant doctors at the hospital. I listened carefully as they told me they thought that I was a very good candidate because I was young and I had not received prior systemic chemother-apy. My disease was still very small, even though it had gone to my bone; the only evident cancer was on my sternum.

Afterward I talked with my oncology team. My oncologist, oncology surgeon, and radiation oncologist gave me the "green light" to go ahead with the trans-plant. My oncologist especially surprised me with her affirmation. She pounded her fist on the table and said, "Georgia, you are going to go in there and suffer and come out cured!"

While driving into the city for this appointment, I had cried and prayed the whole way. I begged the Lord for my life. I told Him that I didn't know what the doc-tors were going to think, but I was willing to do any-thing, whatever it would take, to extend my days. I didn't care how much I would have to suffer. I didn't care what I would have to go through. I just wanted a chance to live.

When my oncologist said, "You will come out cured," I felt God had inspired me through her. I took those words as a confirmation from the Lord that this was the way for me to go. That night, instead of feeling depressed, discouraged, and at a dead end, I felt inspired and invigorated to go ahead with this drastic procedure.

Struggling with My Decision

That evening, Philip and I read the six-page informa-tion sheet about the bone-marrow transplant. It minced no words in describing what the future would hold for me if I chose this radical, experimental treatment.

Mine was to be an autologous bone-marrow transplant, meaning I would donate my own marrow to myself instead of receiving marrow from a donor. During general anesthesia, the doctors would first harvest bone-marrow cells from the hip and freeze them. During the next days to weeks, they would administer very high doses of chemotherapy through a catheter implanted through the skin of the neck in a vein just above the heart. The combination of chemicals used in chemotherapy is toxic to the whole system, killing not only cancerous cells but also all the white blood cells and most of the red blood cells and platelets (small structures that help with blood clotting). The chemicals also cause loss of body and scalp hair, nausea and vomiting, sore mouth and throat (with sores similar to canker sores), diarrhea, fever, sterility, temporary abnormalities in liver function, and more. To compensate for the loss of blood cells, the patient must receive transfusions of red blood cells and platelets from other people.

On the twelfth day after harvesting, the bone marrow is thawed and reinfused into the bloodstream through a catheter. Then the waiting begins . . . waiting to see if the white blood cells will regenerate, which never happens before the tenth day after reinfusion. Unfortunately, the marrow does not always regenerate. When it happens, the first white blood cell count normally shows as 50 to 100 (a normal white count is 4,000 to 6,000). During the wait, the patient has no immune system. Even a small infection can easily cause major complications and sometimes death. Twenty percent of the people who begin this treatment die in the midst of it. More die of later infections or cancer that wasn't killed by the chemotherapy.

We stared at the last page that required our signatures. How could we sign, knowing it could drastically shorten my life?

Philip hesitated. He was torn between the two unknowns. Would I be cured by this radical treatment, or would it push me over the edge and kill me? Uncertainty. Numbing fear.

My firm decision and confidence waned a bit because I didn't know of anybody who had undergone a successful bone-marrow transplant.

When Barbara had received her transplant, her disease had already progressed much further than mine. I hoped that, if I went in at an earlier stage, maybe the transplant would work for me even though it had not worked for Barbara. As with all failed transplant patients, her disease was now spreading *more* rapidly than it would have otherwise because her weakened immune system could not fight the multiplying cancer cells.

The more I considered the treatment, the more desperate I became to find someone who had lived through the bone-marrow transplant and was in successful remission. My mother has a friend whose daughter-in-law, Christine, had just gone through a bone-marrow transplant. I thought, *Oh good! I can call Christine on the phone and ask her how she's doing and what it was like.* When I made the call, her husband, John, answered the phone. I asked to talk to Christine.

"Didn't you hear about her?" John asked.

"Yes, I heard that she had a bone-marrow transplant."

"Right," he replied, "but didn't you hear that she died?"

Of course I hadn't heard. I extended my condolences and hung up the phone. My heart sank to my feet. *O dear Lord,* I prayed. *Here I'm planning to go through with this outrageous procedure, and the only people I know who have done it are Barbara, who is dying, and Christine, who is already dead after only two months.*

That night was very hard to get through. I felt so discouraged, thinking, *Am I doing the right thing? I don't have any encouraging examples.* Yet somehow my spirit was leading me—even thrusting me—in this direction. I kept remembering what my doctor had said about going in and finding my cure, and I was aware of the prayers of so many people that supported me at that moment.

I had to believe that the transplant was my destined path. But at this point I had to choose this path completely by faith. Nothing I could hold on to or see was a positive example. I had to believe that I would go through this fearful procedure and come out on the other side alive. And I had to believe that I was going to come out not only alive but also cured—or at least with a good remission.

As I weighed the options in my mind, I felt the bone-marrow transplant was my only chance for survival and possible cure. The treatment was radical, but the disease was worse. I felt like Tarzan in a movie, with natives chasing me toward a river full of crocodiles. The cancer (like the natives) was going to kill me—and very soon. The treatment (like the river full of crocodiles) was dangerous but was my only hope for escape. I had to dive in.

I decided: "I am going for the cure." We signed the release.

8

Preparing for the Bone-Marrow Transplant

The transplant procedure started in the hospital under general anesthesia. With large needles inserted into my hip bones, the doctors extracted two pints of bone marrow and then froze it. Preserved by cold and chemicals, the marrow awaited the day it would be reinfused into my body. It was eerie to think that my "life" was contained in two pints of bone marrow stored away in some freezer at the hospital. After being in the hospital for a couple of days, I was sent home to recuperate for a few days before returning to the hospital for a six-week stay. During those days at home I sometimes imagined, *What if they lose my bone marrow? What if they get it mixed up with someone else's? I'll be dead!*

Support from My Church and Other Christians

Each person who has a bone-marrow transplant must receive many platelet transfusions and needs someone to serve as a coordinator of blood donors. As I wondered who to ask, I thought of Jane, a friend from my church. I needed her help to find thirty people willing to have their blood checked to determine if their blood platelets would match mine. If they did have a match, they would need to go to the hospital and donate their blood, which would be used for my platelet transfusions. This is not a simple procedure like donating blood in the usual way. Platelet donors must sit in a chair for about three hours with one plastic needle in each arm while a machine separates the platelets from the whole blood and then reinfuses the remainder of the blood back into the donor. Jane agreed to accept the task of coordinating these donors. She found thirty willing people, ten of whom qualified as platelet donors.

Many members from my church were extremely supportive through prayers, cards, meals, and sensitive fellowship. The publishing house where my husband works was also very supportive. Some people came in to work early every day to pray for me. Many of my music teacher colleagues in the area prayed for me and asked their churches to pray for me. Many of my piano students and their parents also prayed for me. And all of my family on my side and on my husband's side were helpful in every way possible. My mother, Joan, and my mother-in-law, Dottie, came to help out in our home every time I had to go into the hospital. They were wonderful "fill-in" moms during all the times I was gone. Many of my high-school and college friends sent me letters of support, and some let me know they had asked their churches to pray for me. Both my grandmother, Ann, and Philip's grandmother, Dorothy, carried me in their hearts and in prayer.

There is no way I could have had such enormous faith at this critical time without the prayers of so many people. I thank God for those who prayed for me.

Their prayers energized me as I went in for the bone-marrow transplant, and their prayers sustained me. I was able to say what the apostle Paul said in the New Testament: "I know that as you pray for me, and as the Holy Spirit helps me, this is all going to turn out for my good" (Philippians 1:19).

My Mental Health

Thirteen months after my diagnosis of breast cancer, I went to the hospital for my bone-marrow transplant. Within that thirteen-month period I had undergone five surgeries and six weeks of radiation treatment. I was exhausted. It was not good for me to be so run-down prior to this major procedure. Concerned that I wouldn't be ready for the trauma, I started to see a psychologist at the hospital who deals with cancer patients. Because he was kind and understanding when I opened my heart and disclosed to him my fears and anxieties, I felt that I had a friend at the hospital.

Both my psychologist and my surgeon were aware of my crazy sense of humor, and they readily accepted my jokes about myself, the hospital, and my treatment. It was good to have some people I could laugh with and who would laugh along with my crazy quips. During one of my pretreatment sessions, I told my psychologist I was worried about "going over the deep end."

"Georgia," he responded, "if you could imagine yourself 'cracking up,' how do you think you would do it? How do you think you would try to cope?"

"I would fantasize," I told him.

"What kind of fantasy?"

"I would keep myself happy by becoming a totally different character. Maybe I would fantasize I was Martha Washington. Of course, that might make me very unhappy. What if I was pretending to be Martha Washington, and George never came to see me? Then I'd really be sad!" I added, "I might also fantasize that I was giving piano concerts in my room."

The psychologist responded, "Well, if the nurses tell me you're charging people admission to come hear your concerts, then I'll be concerned!"

Shaving Off My Hair

Two days before my admission to the bone-marrow transplant unit, I decided to do something drastic about my hair. I knew I would become bald like Kojak as the result of the chemotherapy. To spare myself the humiliation of having all my nice long blonde hair falling out while in the hospital, I decided to have a defrocking party and cut it off myself.

I invited some of my friends to bring their scissors and join me at the beauty salon for this occasion. My friend Elizabeth videotaped the entire event, which instead of being sad turned out to be quite a party. My friends took turns lopping off a big chunk of hair with their scissors until my new hairstyle was an inch long all over my head.

During the process, we laughed and sang the theme to *Hair*, a popular musical from the sixties. When it was time to try on wigs, I decided to purchase something unconventional—a long, platinum-blonde wig. If I had to have an abnormal experience, I might as well go all the way and get that one!

No sooner had I walked into my house and dropped my purse and car keys on the table when the phone rang. A friendly voice from the photography studio said, "I'm just calling to remind you of your five-thirty appointment for your family portrait."

"Thank you," I said, trying to sound polite rather than a cross between horrified and hysterical. I hung up the phone thinking, *I can't believe it! I forgot all about it. Here I just got all my hair cut off, and we have to go in for a family portrait.*

I called the children in from playing outside and said, "Well, boys, we're going to get our photo taken in half an hour. Do you want me to go like this, with my 'buzz,' or do you want me to wear my new Dolly Parton wig?"

They just laughed and said, "You look ridiculous both ways, Mom." But the general consensus was that I should put on my new wig for the family portrait. So we had our photo taken, and everyone managed to smile, even though no one really felt like it. We went out to dinner afterward and tried to have a pleasant family time. But try as we might, everyone was tense and anxious about the impending separation.

Saying Good-bye to My Family

As the day drew closer, I tried not to let my emotions get the best of me, nor to allow myself to be weighed down by my family's feelings. Throughout the course of my illness and treatments, I had progressively separated myself emotionally from my family to help ease the pain. This happened even more as the transplant approached. I feared I might not come out alive.

The Monday I went in, Philip and the boys brought me to the hospital. The boys weren't allowed to come into the transplant unit; they had to say good-bye to me in the hall. All three children were crying, and Philip was crying, feeling the pain of the children. Philip knew he could see me every day, but the boys would be kept out except for a few visits. I couldn't handle facing the reality of the possibilities I faced—of never seeing them again, of death, of the painful, unknown process ahead, so instead I reacted very much like a teenager. I happily said good-bye to my children and told them, "I love you. I'll see you on Sunday when you come to see me." Then I totally turned myself off to how they felt and how I felt.

Chewing my bubble gum, I went to my room and turned my thoughts to fixing my wig for the day and to my new compact-disc stereo that I had brought to the hospital with me. I had received quite a few CDs as gifts from many friends, and I was excited about listening to my new music.

I put myself into a different world, one that was separate from the world of reality and family. I imagined myself to be a totally different person, someone young and buoyant, like a teenager who had just gone away to college and was decorating her dorm room. I covered my wall with posters to cheer me up—ballet dancers, musicians, and pictures of my children and family. Since my hospital stay might be as long as two months, I wanted to make my room an expression of myself, and I wanted to feel like I could still do things that made me happy. Thus—even though it was extravagant and out of the ordinary—I ordered a large electronic piano to be delivered to my room. My husband's grandmother graciously helped me purchase this keyboard, which was delivered the same day I was admitted. This gift was her way of cheering me on and letting me know that she was behind me all the way.

My First Night

From the first night in the hospital, I excelled in denial. I refused to wear hospital clothes and wore my own instead. Wearing a hospital gown seemed to me like succumbing to the role of victim. I never wanted to be just a patient; I wanted to retain my own self-identity and dignity. I brought nice clothes, pretty gowns, and bathrobes so that, while I knew I would be looking ugly, I could try and make myself as pretty as possible.

That evening, after answering all the medical questions and filling out all the forms, I started playing my electronic piano. Many doctors, nurses, and residents heard that there was this lady in her room playing music. No one would have imagined from my behavior that I would be starting such a hideous procedure the next day. This was both sad and funny, but I thought, *If I'm going to die of this procedure I want to have a good time before I die.* So I invited people into my room, played jazz and classical music, and led sing-alongs. We partied, and whoever came along joined the party.

After everyone left that night, one of the nurses came by and asked if I would go down the hall to visit a lady named Colette, who had come in to have her bone marrow harvested. Colette and I had much in common. We were the same age, we both had three boys, and we both had breast cancer. I talked to Colette for about an hour and tried to encourage her in her fight against cancer. Over the next year, Colette and I became close friends. I'm grateful I met her that first night. Not only was it a great distraction, it was the beginning of a genuine relationship in which we helped each other in our struggle to survive.

Chapter

9

The Big Blast

The first morning, a nurse named Julie came into my room with the first round of chemotherapy. The chemicals were in a large plastic bag. As I looked at that container of poison—megadoses of thiotepa, cisplatin, and cytoxin—tears fell down my cheeks. I was so scared. Once that bag was empty, I couldn't turn back. I hated having to be in the position where I had been dealt such difficult choices.

My husband, sitting next to me, held one of my hands, and Julie held the other. Then Julie, a born-again Christian, began to pray. "Thank You, Lord, that modern medicine has developed to the point where we can do this procedure—a bone-marrow transplant—to try to beat the cancer. I pray that You would direct the chemotherapy to every cancer cell and that every single cell would be destroyed. Thank You, Lord, for Your life. I pray that much life and much grace and much supply of the Holy Spirit would be ministered to Georgia right now."

As I continued to cry, my tears of fear were transformed into tears of peace and thanksgiving. I saw Julie as a channel of God's grace. I felt her own compassion and kindness, and I trusted in her knowledge as a nurse. I saw the chemotherapy as a product of human genius through which God would dispense His grace. On my nightstand next to my bed there was a Bible, and on my other side was my husband. And God's presence was in the room. Everything I needed was right there with me. I told Julie to go ahead and begin the chemotherapy. Listening to some beautiful music in the background, I closed my eyes and went off into dreamland—thinking about my children and about my life when I would get out of the hospital. It was a very peaceful, calm time. I attribute this to the supply of the Spirit and the reassurance of Julie and Philip.

At this moment, Philip later told me, he believed that God was going to use the medicine to cure me. He had hoped that God would heal me directly, but that had not happened. Now he realized that divine intervention would come with medical intervention. He wrote a poem to capture the moment:

> *you lie in bed*
> *I sit by you*
> *squeezing your hand*
> *as I look*
> *at a Gideon Bible*
> *on your bedstand*
> *and a nurse quietly working*
> *with a machine*
> *pumping chemotherapy*
> *into your veins—*
> *we all sense*
> *His presence*

over all
and feel
no contradiction

march 16, 1990
my wife's first day of chemotherapy

Dealing with Isolation, Physical Mutilation, and Dementia

Patients in the bone-marrow transplant unit are kept in isolation because their immune systems have been destroyed by the strong chemotherapy, making them susceptible to any kind of infection. Consequently, the patient spends a lot of time alone. This isolation is dreadful for a gregarious person like me. Philip and I decided ahead of time that he would spend most of his time outside of work with the children, so I spent many lonely hours in the hospital. Often I was unaware of isolation because I was on so many drugs. When I was aware, the evenings were the most difficult. That's when I spent a lot of time calling on the Lord, praying and dealing with all the desperate feelings that I had. I fought to overcome my loneliness, the fear of dying, and my rapidly degenerating physical appearance.

My short hair fell out within a week. I tried not to look at myself in the mirror when I went to the bathroom; it was too shocking to see myself totally bald. To make matters worse, the large doses of antibiotics given to control internal infections caused severe skin rashes. Furthermore, I bruised very easily because my platelet count was so low. From head to toe I was bruised, and my eyes were bloodshot. I looked like a little monster, as did many people in the bone-marrow transplant unit. I had a hard time picturing myself the way I used to look, but I did my best to imagine myself restored from head to toe.

I couldn't take any food by mouth for one month because the large doses of chemotherapy wreaked havoc on my gastrointestinal system. I couldn't digest food or even hold it down. Every night a nurse would bring a bag of liquid food and feed it into my catheters while I slept. I was so excited when I finally could have a Popsicle and a cup of tea. I felt like a little child eating a brand-new treat.

The combination of drugs—chemotherapy, antibiotics, drugs to help me tolerate daily blood transfusions and other side effects of treatment—caused me to be psychologically demented. For about a month, when I tried to watch television I couldn't understand what was going on. On one occasion I got excited because I finally understood what I was seeing on TV. As I watched a golf game in process, I said, "Oh, yes, I see. They're going to hit the ball, and then they're going to follow the ball, and they're going to try to get it into a hole. It's a game of golf." I felt like I was coming back to the real world because I could understand what was going on.

Sometimes, when medical staff and others would inadvertently communicate that they expected me to die, I would remind myself that I was doing this to live. Sometimes when I felt physically, emotionally, or spiritually assaulted, I would repeat to myself, "Live, live, live."

There is a saying in the Bible, "As a man thinks, so is he." My situation was very difficult physically, but I would fight against it with all my mind, realizing that tomorrow might be a better day. I tried not to be afraid to disclose my fears, anxieties, and pains to the doctors and the nurses. I found the nurses and doctors in the transplant unit to be very encouraging. And when I felt that my bad days would never end, they assured me that better days would come. And they were right.

Love from Family and Friends

Every night around seven-thirty I called home to talk to my family. I asked my children what they had eaten for dinner, if they had finished their homework, if they had watched a TV show, and what they were doing with their friends. Sometimes it was a very short conversation, but it was very important to the boys and myself to say to each other, "I love you. Have a good night. We'll talk tomorrow."

My parents were extremely helpful during this time. It pained them deeply to see their beloved daughter suffer so much. My father, George, agonized for me because he had lost his sister to breast cancer when she was thirty-two years old. My mother, Joan, hid her pain and took care of my children with a positive spirit.

I received many telephone calls from my parents, my husband's parents, my sister, my brothers, my brothers-in-law, my sisters-in-law, and my friends. For quite a while I was so choked up to hear their voices that I could hardly respond. Whatever they would say to me I would answer, "I know."

For example, my sister Sally would say, "I love you, Dorda" (the name she called me ever since she could talk).

"I know," I responded. And then I would cry.

My sister is my soul mate. She buoyed me up on a daily basis with telephone calls and cards. She also had many of her friends in New York City cheering me on.

I was fortunate to receive hundreds of cards and letters. Every day I received at least eight cards and letters from people all over the place—even from people I didn't know. These were inspiring letters and hope-filled messages from many friends and family members. My daily stack of mail was a great source of encouragement, comfort, and inspiration. Even so, I would often cry as I read my mail. It was a very emotional time for me because I deeply sensed the love of God and the ministry of the church.

I soaked in the support from God's people through telephone calls, letters, and notes. I cherished this visible ministry. And the invisible prayer ministry was just as constant. I was daily supplied by the Spirit and the prayers of many believers. I am eternally grateful for those who were so faithful to pray for me.

Compassionate Care

The first doctor who took care of me in the bone-marrow transplant unit was a compassionate man. When he made his daily rounds he would hold my hand and talk to me in detail about my medical condition. He gave me his undivided attention and answered all my questions, from the trite to the critical. Furthermore, he, as a lover of the musical arts, talked with me about the opera and other musical performances. It was wonderful to have a doctor who not only was compassionate and brilliant but who linked me to the life I lived before I came into the hospital.

One of my night nurses, Jean, was a very caring Christian. Every night she had to awaken me to give me medication or a transfusion of blood platelets. I was usually very groggy because I would take a sleeping pill around eleven at night, so I didn't speak with her very much. But when I woke up in the morning and went into the bathroom, I would find a Bible verse waiting for me. I knew Jean had been there the night before. She always wrote an encouraging psalm or verse—something that would strengthen my hope and trust in the Lord.

The hospital psychologist also came in just about every day to see me. He held my hand and let me know he was there for me. I could depend on his daily visits, and if I ever felt like I was "losing it," he would come and help me gain perspective on the situation.

I depended on the competence, care, and wisdom of my doctors, the care and encouragement from the nurses, the care of my psychologist, the devotion of my husband and family members, the concern of my friends who loved me, the care of my friends who nourished me spiritually, and the mutual care that I developed with other patients who were also fighting for their life. And most of all, I depended on the Great Physician, Jesus Christ. We are not alone in this life. When we ask for help, many people show their love and concern.

The Gift of Blood

The people who came to the hospital to donate blood platelets usually wanted to stop by and say hello to me. This helped me associate the donated platelets with the donors themselves. So when I received a blood transfusion, I tried to think of it as a love offering given to me by one of these people—not just as something that would make me violently sick! I got the "rigors" (violent shaking) and fevers. But I had to have this blood for my survival, so I took it as a gift of love. I realized it was a sacrifice for people to come into the city and sit there for three hours and give blood for me. And I learned that many of these donors spent that time praying for me.

This made me think of the Lord Jesus. He shed His blood for us so that we would have life. As I lay there, I would thank the Lord for giving His blood for me. The blood of Jesus became extremely precious to me. It had been precious before, but it took on a new dimension of preciousness—like a diamond seen in new light. Jesus was God—God who became a man and shed His blood for us that we might have life. This renewed understanding was so sweet, even though I was feeling terribly sick. The sweet Spirit of the risen Christ was with me, and I reflected on what Jesus did to give us eternal life.

Life out of Death

The process of poisoning my body with chemotherapy
to kill all the cancer cells brought me very close to the
death I was trying to avoid. The doctors hoped by now
every cancer cell had been eliminated and that I could
survive all the coming days during which I would be
without an immune system. On the twelfth day, they
reinfused my thawed bone marrow into my catheter.
Now it was time for all of us to watch and wait for the
white blood cells to regenerate. The doctors cautioned
that the earliest show of white blood cells would be on
the tenth day, and that even then it might still be as low
as 50 to 100 white cells.

Without an immune system, my body could not
fight even the smallest infection. I developed an infection of unknown source during this time without an
immune system. For nine days I was deliriously ill with
a fever spiking 104.5 degrees daily. On the afternoon of
the ninth day, the doctor on rotation spoke quietly in
the hallway with Philip. "I need to be honest with you.
Your wife's life is in danger right now. If this fever
doesn't break . . ."

Philip panicked at her words. He knew my vital

organs couldn't take such a high fever much longer. The doctor's words broke into his frightened thoughts. "We're preparing a refrigerated bed to put Georgia on if her temperature does not come down by morning."

Lord, You died for her, now live for her! Philip prayed.

He called several people to ask if they would pray for me. On that Wednesday evening, the word spread to many people and many churches that I was in a life-threatening situation. That night, as many church groups gathered for prayer, many people prayed for me. Philip also spent most of the night in prayer for me. In desperation he prayed again and again, *Lord, You died for her, now live for her!*

I also prayed by saying, "Live, live, live." I repeated this over and over and quoted a verse from the Bible: "With his stripes we are healed" (Isaiah 53:5, KJV). I had said that verse to myself many times during my illness, but now I desperately claimed it for nearly twenty-four hours without ceasing because I knew I was on the verge of death. I just kept claiming, "With His stripes I am healed."

As I claimed this truth and felt its reality in my life, I deeply appreciated the sufferings of Jesus. Even though we know Jesus is God, Jesus was also fully man, with the same muscle fiber and nerve endings and all the body parts that can hurt—and most of my body parts were hurting very badly at this time. I felt as though I participated in the sufferings of Jesus Christ and better understood His sufferings. He had stripes because He was beaten. I knew He felt each lashing inflicted on His body before His crucifixion. His nerve endings were just like my nerve endings, and His pain—although more severe—was like my pain. On behalf of all of us, He took our pain and He died our death so that we might have life!

I knew how many drugs I had been given—the large doses of toxic chemicals and all the antibiotics that were given to sustain me. I thought of all the surgeries and all the radiation treatments I had endured. I realized that all of them were an attempt to heal me. But my deepest and truest realization was "With His stripes I am healed." Even though I had taken everything that modern medicine could offer, I was fully aware that if I was going to be healed I needed to glorify God for His Son, Jesus Christ, who became our sin offering by being brutally murdered.

As I went to sleep late into the night, I continued to repeat quietly, "With His stripes you are healed."

An Honest Prayer from John

Philip had sent the boys away to be with relatives in California for spring vacation for the week after my bone marrow was transfused. On that critical ninth day, they returned yet were unable to see me. My twelve-year-old son, John, with his fists clenched by his side, approached his father and in extreme frustration said, "I want you to buy me some boxing gloves!"

"Why?"

"Because I just want to hit anything and everything. I'm so mad," John explained.

"Who are you mad at?" his dad asked.

"I'm mad at God. I'm mad at the devil. I'm mad

at Mom. I'm mad at the whole world! Why couldn't some dork mom get cancer? Why did *my* mom have to get cancer and go through all this?"

His dad then said, "If you're mad, let's talk to God about it."

"I already have. It doesn't do any good."

"Well, let's try again. I understand how you feel. And I don't have all the answers right now. But I know that Mom really needs us to pray for her."

So John agreed to pray.

"Do you want to repeat my words?"

"No. I'll pray on my own."

John bowed his head, then spoke clearly and directly: "Jesus, the Bible says You are real. My dad says You are real. But I don't know if You are real. I want You to prove You are real by healing Mom."

Hearing this, his father burst into tears. He thought, *Lord, You are really on the spot now! Are You going to break his heart? Oh please, hear his prayer!*

Life out of Death!

When I woke up the next morning, I saw my wonderful night nurse, Jean.

Excitedly she asked, "Georgia, guess what? Your fever's down. It's 98.7! And," she added, her smile taking over her whole face, "you have a white count!"

Wow! For a bone-marrow transplant patient, having a white count was like a person on a desert island getting a cup of fresh water—a matter of life or death. I had to trust that all those bone-marrow cells would know where to go when they were reinfused into my body. That they would go "home" by themselves. I had to trust that the freezing process hadn't killed the cells. I had to trust that they would replenish, propagate, and grow. Once this happened, my own bone marrow would regenerate new white blood cells and other blood cells.

And now the verdict was in. I had a white count, and the count was a phenomenal 700! No one would have guessed that after such a difficult infection the white blood cells would manifest themselves on the earliest possible day, nor that they would come charging in like cavalry instead of trickling in like shy newcomers. This was a sign that my transplant had actually worked and that I was going to live!

I lifted up my hands, started crying, rejoicing, and praising the Lord. I knew the prayers had been answered. The battle had been won. I had survived the bone-marrow transplant!

My tears flowed and flowed. I kept thanking Jesus. I thanked God. I thanked the Spirit. I thanked the angels. I thanked anyone I knew who had anything to do with this. My cup was overflowing. Even though I still felt terribly sick, my spirit and my soul strongly rejoiced in the Lord. I was so grateful to all the people who had been praying. And I felt relieved, like a prizefighter walking out of the ring beat up but relieved that the fight was over and had been won.

Sharing the Good News

I wanted to tell Philip right away. I knew he would be calling me to find out how I was doing so that he could take the report to the people he worked with who would be praying for me that morning. But I couldn't wait for him to call me.

With tears of joy I said, "Honey, I can't believe it; my fever's down. And I have a white count of 700!"

He started crying and rejoicing at the same time—full of emotion. He was ecstatic. In his ecstasy, he exploded with praise and joyful thanksgiving, shouting, "Hallelujah! Hallelujah! Praise the Lord!" We exulted together.

After I talked to Philip, he immediately shared the news with the boys. Relief and joy spread through them all—especially John, for now he believed in the Lord who had answered his prayer.

My dear friend and neighbor, Carol, drove John to school that day. She later told us that John had changed into a sunshine child. She couldn't get over the difference between his new outlook that day and the way he had been all the other days she had driven him. He had been so depressed and weighed down with care and anxiety.

The news got around quickly that day: "Georgia is going to live!" It was a day of rejoicing—for me and for those who prayed to our Lord to spare my life.

> *as I watched her life*
> *hang in the balance*
> *and felt the weight of death*
> *I begged the Arbiter*
> *to lift the burden*
> *and restore her wasted health.*
> *I asked Him who died for her*

to live for her
and call the marrow
and tomorrow into being.

He must have heard the spirit
of a thousand warring prayers
rushing through the air
to His throne of grace,
for He made the grafted host multiply
to form a cellular force
against the insidious enemy—
germ fought germ in fervent battle
until the fever lifted.

what moved His hand to tip the scale
is not clear to me or visible.
was it the praying saints or the awful fevers?
was it the thought of children without a mother?
she was touched, though, with heaven's grace
and given glory's extra weight.
she sprang to life
and I rose up to praise
the God of mercy.

After Death Comes Resurrection

With successful transplantation of my own healthy bone marrow back into my sick and weakened body, I had confidence that I had reached the other side of the crocodile-infested waters. I had been brought to the brink of death. Indeed, I had hovered over the precipice and was now on my way back to life. But the way would not be easy and was filled with indescribable misery. The horrible side effects listed by the protocol and consent sheet Philip and I had signed seized me with full force. I had never felt so horrible. I had a skin rash from head to toe. I had open sores and my skin itched all over. To add to this agony, I was still bruised all over from not having enough platelets. My white count of 700 plunged, heightening my anxiety and teasing my faith.

Good Friday arrived in the middle of this suffering, a week after my white blood cells began to generate. Jane, who had coordinated my blood donor program, came to see me. When she saw how terrible I looked and how weak I was, she was aghast. I could hardly move or get out of bed. The nine-day fever had taken everything out of me. I was so weak I didn't feel like talking. I lay there listlessly, comforted by Jane's presence. As tears rolled down my cheeks, I nodded or shook my head as Jane gently asked me questions.

She said, "Georgia, do you know what day it is?"

I shook my head side to side on the pillow.

She replied, "Today is Good Friday. This is the day we're remembering the Lord was crucified. I'm sure you can very keenly identify with the death of our Lord."

I nodded.

I felt the presence of the Lord coming through Jane. It slowly filled me, giving me inner spiritual strength. I sensed that Jane deeply and dearly wanted to minister to me. Her sense of compassion, looking at me there so weak and ugly, caused her to have great love for me. She must have known that words were not enough—that somehow I had a deeper need. I could tell that she was groping—trying to determine what to do to meet my needs. She held my hand and talked with me very gently. Then she started crying. With tears streaming down her face, she lay her head on my stomach and then on my legs.

Her compassionate actions reminded me of Mary in the Gospels of Matthew and Luke when she broke her alabaster box and poured the precious ointment on Jesus. And so Jane "broke her alabaster box" and poured the best of her spirit and her soul and her heart onto me. She drew something precious from the deepest part of her soul, realizing that anything less wouldn't have been adequate. I received it as a wonderful ministry—what an incredibly sweet experience!

As we remembered the death of our Lord Jesus

that Good Friday, we both had a strong taste of death because of the others passing near death elsewhere in the transplant unit and because I had just been there myself. Yet we both sensed the sweetness of the death of Jesus Christ. And together we enjoyed the hope of His resurrection, which we would celebrate on Easter. We sensed the hope in Christ and were fortified by His resurrection power.

On Easter I was feeling better. My fluctuating white count had come up to about 1,000—where it would stay for a few days, solidifying my confidence in the success of the procedure. Philip, my boys, and Philip's parents came in to celebrate Easter with me. I was allowed to be with them if I wore a mask, gown, and gloves.

We gathered in a small visiting room, and Philip's father, Richard, led the singing. We sang songs about the resurrection of Christ, we prayed, and we offered thanksgiving. What a sweet, wonderful time we had celebrating the resurrection of Christ. His resurrection meant so much more to us that day because we had all witnessed a resurrection in my life.

Hearing the News of Barbara's Death

After Philip's parents and the boys left that day to go back home, Philip stayed with me. As we talked, I told Philip, "I think we should call and see how Barbara is doing. I wonder if she died. Please call, Philip, and tell me what they say."

Philip responded, "You told me not to let you know, so I didn't. But now you seem to have some strength for the first time, and I feel that you can handle the news. Georgia, Barbara died this past week, and I went to her wake on Thursday."

I started crying and continued to cry as we talked about Barbara. My heart was broken. I missed my dear friend. I didn't get to say good-bye. I thought about the decisions I had made along the way, wondering if they had been the right ones.

While I had been preparing to go into the bone-marrow transplant unit, Barbara had been readmitted to the hospital. The cancer had taken over her liver and had gone to her brain. Our last visit was right before I went in for my transplant. I had really hoped she would be able to visit me while I was going through my treatments. But she got sicker and sicker and wasn't able to come and see me at all. She tried to call me and I tried to call her, but we never got through to one another.

I thought about her the whole time I was in the transplant unit and wondered how she was doing. I knew she was near the end. I had even sensed that she had died, but I was afraid to ask. She was my dearest friend. If I knew for certain she had died, then I would have to struggle even more with the thought that plagued me all along: *I'm next.*

Because of this struggle I had asked Philip not to tell me if Barbara died while I was going through the bone-marrow transplant. I knew that if he told me this, I could get very depressed and wouldn't be able to fight as hard for my life. I had to believe the bone-marrow transplant would work for me even though it hadn't worked for Barbara. So Philip agreed not to tell me until I came out of the hospital or could handle this news.

To encourage me, Philip wanted me to know that he spoke with Barbara's sister-in-law at the funeral home. She told Philip that during the last days of Barbara's life she kept talking about me—what a wonderful friend I was to her and how much I helped her to know the Lord. Barbara kept me in her heart. Even though she was dying, she imagined herself standing with me as I was going through my treatment. She was suffering, she couldn't see me, she couldn't talk to me, but she was talking about me.

Philip explained to me that she had died peacefully. She gathered her family around her just before she died and told them, "I'm going to be with the Lord now. I just want you to understand that I have accepted Jesus Christ as my Savior, and I know where I'm going. I'm going to be with Jesus."

She explained to her family how I had talked with her about the Lord and salvation. So, even though I was grieving terribly about the loss of such a precious friend and wonderful person, I had some comfort in knowing that she believed in the Lord Jesus and knew that she would live with Him eternally.

"Georgia," Philip said, "you gave Barbara the two best gifts a person can give. You gave her true friendship, and you helped her have a relationship with Jesus Christ."

My Last Week in the Hospital

Peter, my youngest son, was to turn eight years old on April 21, about two weeks after Easter. I made it my goal to get out of the hospital in time for Peter's birthday. I hoped I would stabilize enough to be taken off all the antibiotics, to not need any more blood transfusions, and to eat better on my own—as well as to learn how to take care of my catheter by myself. All of these were prerequisites for being dismissed from the hospital. But on April 21, I was still in the hospital. So Peter's birthday party came to me!

All three of my boys along with Philip and his parents came to the hospital, bringing with them Coke and pizza. We had a party in the same little visiting room where we had enjoyed our Easter service. Although I could barely taste that the Coke was really Coca-Cola and the pizza was really pizza, it was still a fun day. The pizza and Coke were much better than hospital food! And nothing could beat the joy of being there with my boys.

Toxicity

I couldn't leave the hospital when I wanted to because my skin was having violent toxic reactions to all the chemicals and antibiotics that had been pumped into my body. For many days I was on ten antibiotics at once. And nearly every time I was given a blood transfusion or blood platelets, my system reacted negatively. Eventually my skin developed what is called a "toxic eruption." I was already bruised from head to toe, and then I had this skin eruption from head to toe. I looked like a monster and felt miserable. I anxiously wanted to get out of the hospital to attempt some sort of normal life.

I could see it was sunny and beautiful outside. I couldn't stand being inside one more day. But since I had such a terrible rash, they couldn't let me leave until they got it under control. So I had to stay there an extra week—for a total of six weeks.

Reflections before Going Home

In the days before my release, I thought about some of the significant spiritual experiences I had while in the hospital. I had bargained with the Lord to spare my life. In the deep of many nights, I spent the quiet, lonely hours bargaining with the Lord. If He would please spare me from death, I would serve Him and live my life for Him when I got out. And I begged Him, "Please let me live. I promise You, I will not forget the suffering people of the earth. I will not forget the people who are devastated by cancer. And especially—I will befriend those women who have had a bone-marrow transplant. I want to give them hope and encouragement and be an example of one who made it through. I promise You, Lord, that I will do whatever You want me to do. And I will be a testimony of Your life."

Giving God the Glory

I honored my bargain to God even before I left the hospital. The first people I witnessed to were my nurses and doctors. I told them, "It was not only modern medicine that brought me through; it was the power of God."

I didn't want to underestimate the value of the doctors and the nurses and modern medical technologies, but I wanted them to see that I lived through this radical treatment because God sustained my life. I told my psychologist, doctors, nurses, and other staff members that Jesus was with me and was my true Healer. Some of them said, "Amen." But others said, "Well, we don't know what to attribute your turn for the best to, but it's good that it happened." And there were other noncommittal responses.

I didn't care if they thought I was crazy. I wanted to give the glory to the Lord.

My final week in the hospital brought out thoughts about how my sufferings had changed my thinking about life. Of course, I hate suffering of any kind, but this suffering helped me clarify my priorities. While in the depth of my agony, I never lost the focus that if I did live, my chief purpose was to be a vessel for the Lord, to do His will. I knew that I would have never chosen this path—to experience a terminal illness, to fight like a crazy person for my life, and to almost die in the process of seeking a cure. But since it had been my path, I wanted the Lord to be able to use what I had gained through this experience. I realized that my top priority was to be a testimony for the Lord. I, a fallen sinner saved by grace, was actually being transformed by the Lord's life. If there is any good in me I have to attribute it to the life-saving power of Christ. My number one purpose for my days left on earth was to manifest His marvelous life.

Furthermore, I realized that my purpose was to be faithful to my husband and my three sons. My career was definitely third on the list of priorities, my social life was fourth, and anything else came after these. This didn't mean that I would be limited to living my life for Philip and the boys, but it meant I should give them my best affection and direct my energies toward them. They were the ones I was living for. I had new joy thinking about being in my kitchen, serving meals to my sons and husband.

Leaving Some Dear Friends

I couldn't wait to leave the hospital, even though I knew I would leave behind some dear friends. Of all the friends I made there, Rob and Ellen and their little boy, Ryan, who was there for a bone-marrow transplant, made the most lasting impression. Ryan was only two-and-a-half years old. He had a rare childhood cancer called neuroblastoma. These parents had spent nearly the whole year before I met them living in Children's Hospital with their son. They watched him go through surgeries, radiation treatment, and chemotherapy—none of which worked. The bone-marrow transplant was the last effort to try to save Ryan's life.

Many times when I felt rock-bottom miserable, I would take a walk down the corridor and see little Ryan. He had balloons in his hand, little Nike tennis shoes on his feet, a baseball cap on his head, a mask over his face, and a gown covering his body. It humbled me to see him. I understood my disease and why I had to suffer to get rid of it, while little Ryan (who was just as miserable as I was) had no understanding of what was going on. My heart went out to him and to his parents. How awful to watch your child suffer so. I am sure his parents would rather have suffered in his stead. Whenever I saw Rob and Ellen, we would try to encourage one another. And then we would try to make Ryan laugh a little bit.

Rob and Ellen were very good to me. They wondered, knowing how they loved their son, how I could tolerate the last couple of years being separated from my sons so much. So we had a very sweet camaraderie—especially Ellen and I. I would tell her about the strength that comes in Christ and the faith that we can have in the Lord Jesus Christ—and how His Spirit is tireless when we are so weary and exhausted. I would tell her that there is One we can depend on, One who can give us a tireless spirit. She would also buoy me up with the same fellowship.

Our fellowship continued when I left the hospital. I grieved with her when Ryan died. His memory is in our hearts, and he is with the Lord. Happily, Ellen became pregnant and gave birth to another son. I rejoiced with her for this fresh beginning.

13

Going Home

The pure, clean bone-marrow unit wrapped a protective cocoon around me for six weeks, keeping me safe from the germs and bacteria of the outside world. Then, on a lovely spring day—April 26, the forty-second day of my hospitalization—the doctor said I could go home. As I packed my cards, rolled up my posters, and folded my robes and nightgowns, I thought of the new life reborn in that room. The pain. The joy. The fear. The hours and hours of solitude. I looked forward to going home, happy to get out of "the pit." After all, a butterfly can only stay in a cocoon for so long. Then it's time to try to fly on her own.

But plans to go home also frightened me. My fragile, newborn immune system could easily contract any infection and land me right back in the hospital. And going home meant a household with three boys, two dogs, and who-knows-what kind of germs in the house—as well as facing the rest of the real world with all its bacterial surprises.

Each of my nurses came in before I left to say good-bye and to admonish me, "Make sure you wear your mask in the house, around your children, and any-where else there are people. And you must wash your hands many times a day."

After packing the CDs and stereo, I dressed care-fully, thinking of my boys and their reaction to my ghastly appearance. I attempted to hide my all-over bruising and skin rash beneath a nice dress. I covered my bald head with the crazy platinum wig I had pur-chased on defrocking day. Nothing could hide my bloodshot eyes.

As I walked to the car, I shielded my eyes from the bright sunny day. The end of April didn't know many days as hot as this one. I eased myself into the car, where still heat had been baking the insides. I unrolled the window, hoping the heat would escape enough for comfort. Yet even after the car began to move, the air rushing inside didn't help. The wig sat on my head trapping the heat next to my scalp, prickling and stick-ing in unbearable discomfort.

"Philip, I have to take this wig off. It's just too hot." Without waiting for him to answer, I swept the wig off my head. Instant relief!

As I settled back into my seat to savor the ride home and to think about all that awaited me there—new freedoms, new fears—I noticed that my head was getting all kinds of attention. As people drove by, they did drastic double takes. I told myself, *You'd better get used to this.* I realized there were many hot days ahead when I wouldn't want to wear something on my head, and I knew I was going to be stared at.

Breaking the Ice

When we arrived home, I could hear the boys yelling as their excitement spilled out the open windows and spread out to the car. "Mom's home! Mom's home!"

Philip opened the front door for me, and I stepped in. The boys' excitement vanished, replaced by gaping mouths. Their astonishment over the rash and bald head didn't surprise me. I could tell by the looks on their faces that they wanted to be positive and not hurt my feelings. Although they had seen me on visits to the hospital, they could not hide their shock at how I looked. I had always worn my wig to protect them from my ghastly appearance.

I knew it was up to me to break the ice and help them feel more comfortable. So I cast my best "stern mother" look at them and said, "Now look, you guys. I've been through a real ordeal and I'm tired. So I want you to stay out of my hair!"

All three faces broke into laughter. "But Mom!" they howled, "You don't have any hair!"

That did it. From then on, they felt safe joking about my appearance. Peter even told me, "You should get a job on the TV show 'Aliens!'"

Rediscovering My Identity

My mother, Joan, who came to take care of the boys while I was in the bone-marrow transplant unit, wanted to come and help me after my return home. I declined her generous offer, wanting to adjust to being a family again by ourselves.

More than anything else, I needed time alone. The

traumatic events of the past fourteen months had not only buried my identity but had drastically changed it. The intensified struggle altered my perspective on life and even my personality. During the nonstop treatments, I had been like Gunga Din, Geronimo, and Rocky. In all my life I never had to fight for so long without any reprieve.

And now that I was to get a break, I needed to find the real Georgia Comfort—a person with real feelings, hopes, and dreams. But what were they? The only way to find out was to spend time with myself. I gained that time during the day while the boys were in school. Women from the church brought dinner for the first two weeks, so I did not have to worry about feeding my family.

After my return home, I not only suffered the emotional and physical results of the transplant itself, but the enormous doses of chemotherapy had induced premature menopause. I soon found myself floundering from the effects of this also: hot flashes, night sweats, mood swings—everything all at once. Emotionally I was disoriented day to day; it was difficult to grasp what had happened and what continued to happen to my body.

My Husband's Love

The mirror was my enemy. For the first few weeks after my return home, any glance in the mirror drew attention to the ghastly creature I had become, reminding me that my femininity had been assaulted. I cried each time I saw the creature with a bald head, bloodshot eyes, bruised skin, and rashes erupting all over. A two-pronged Hickman catheter, connected to a vein, hung from my neck. My left breast implant had somehow deformed and floated up my chest. No other woman I knew had one breast up and one down. I looked hideous. How could I accept this aberration as me?

Philip was a crucial element to the emotional healing that needed to take place. Early in our marriage, he had focused his energies on pursuing his education and career. His interests, pursuits, and desires had taken precedence over mine. Yet from the onset of my illness, a tremendous switch took place. He put me first, ahead of his needs and desires.

Philip would come home at lunchtime to support me, encourage me, and help me change the dressing on the catheter. He held me while I cried in his arms. Again and again we'd have the same conversation. "Philip, I hate myself. I hate this creature I've become. I hate how I look. I hate that I don't know who or what I am."

"Georgia," he would softly reply, "You are my beautiful girl. I remember . . ." Then he would describe the qualities that had attracted him to me so many years ago. His love and compassion poured into my soul, seeing beyond the pathetic, ugly image to something beautiful. He talked of how I would look after my recovery. Then, with a gentle touch, he said, "You are beautiful because you are alive."

C h a p t e r

14

An Alien in My Own World

The children, having adjusted to my baldness, didn't mind if I went around the house without my scarf on. But while they accepted me for who I was, they were very self-conscious around their friends. They wanted to make sure I had either my wig or scarf on, so they wouldn't be embarrassed.

When their friends came to the house, my kids gave me the red alert: "Mom, put your scarf on! Jason's at the door." Or they warned me earlier in the day: "Mom, make sure you have your scarf on after school. Chad is coming over."

One day, however, I had forgotten to put something on my head when I answered the door for one of Jeremy's friends. He stood frozen, his brown eyes widening as big as saucers. "Mrs. Comfort?" he stammered.

"Yes," I answered calmly. Then I realized—*Oh, my goodness—here I am answering the door bald-headed.* "I'm sorry," I quickly added. "I just had treatment for cancer."

I ran upstairs and put my scarf on. I returned and chatted with him awhile until he regained his composure.

Unfortunately, this was not an isolated incident.

My bizarre appearance continually made people wonder and made people laugh.

From Another Planet

My son Jeremy has a Siberian husky named Nanook, which he had gotten that year for Christmas. Nanook had a propensity for jumping over the fence and wandering around the neighborhood.

Very early one morning I saw the dog escape. I wrapped myself in my bathrobe, leaving my wig on top of my dresser. I quickly got a piece of salami from the refrigerator, climbed into the car, and drove slowly down the street.

I glanced up and down both sides of the street until I saw the dog coming out from behind someone's house. I stopped the car in front of the house and quietly opened the door.

Oh good, I thought. *No one's outside to see my bald head and bathrobe. I'll call the dog, offer him the salami, he'll jump into the car, and we'll head for home.*

I padded around the car and stood on the sidewalk. "Nanook!" I called softly. "Nanook!" I waved the piece of salami enticingly.

At that moment, I noticed a woman sitting on her porch reading the newspaper. Her wide, startled eyes caught mine. She stared as though she was experiencing a visitation from a being from outer space who spoke a different language.

As she stared at me, Nanook suddenly leapt into the Jeep. I jumped in behind him, slammed the door, and took off down the street.

A chuckle bubbled up inside this alien from Mars. What a ridiculous, hysterical scenario! I would love to have that one on video.

The Weird Lady on the Block

Beginning in May and into the summer, I took a couple of walks every day. Because my skin had been so damaged from all the treatments, I couldn't take any direct sunlight. So when the sun was shining I had to cover myself up from head to toe.

There were some little girls on my street about five and six years old. When they saw me coming down the street on a bright sunny day, my outfit confounded them. Here was a lady who wore clothes that completely covered her body and also wore sunglasses, scarf, and hat—under an umbrella!

They sat by the sidewalk, looked up at me, and said, "Mrs. Comfort, it's a nice day. Why are you carrying an umbrella in the sun? It doesn't make any sense."

Since I couldn't explain to them why I had to be covered up, I just said, "Well, my doctor wants me to do this." I didn't elaborate.

They continued to stare at me and said, "Boy, that's the weirdest thing we've ever seen."

"Flip Your Wig"

Two months after my return home, I ventured to the Great America amusement park with my sons, my neighbor Carol, and her sons. Some of the big attractions at Great America are the giant roller coasters. People stand in long lines to get on the Shock Wave or the American Eagle. Then after the ride they get off, trembling and talking as if it had been designed to kill them! Although I was still too weak to go on roller coasters, I was fascinated by watching them.

The passengers climb into a black vinyl bucket seat, with a U-shaped bar pinning them down so they won't fall out. They hold onto the bar for more security. But ultimately, as they pick up speed, they are at the mercy of the roller-coaster ride. The ups and downs, the jarring turns and swirly swoops. Long uphill climbs before heart-stopping drops. Never knowing what will happen next. Deafened by the machinery, the screaming, and their own fear.

Many times in the course of my cancer treatment I had said to people, "I feel like I'm on a roller coaster." But I didn't want to be on that ride. I didn't ask to be there. I couldn't get off unless I wanted to die. So I held on tight: I wanted to live.

After a long day in the hot sun, I didn't look forward to riding home in a car with a broken air conditioner. All day long I had worn my wig so the children wouldn't feel embarrassed. We hadn't gone far when I said, "Carol, I know your children haven't seen me bald, but I can't stand this wig one more minute. I'm having hot flashes, and I'm miserable."

She shrugged her shoulders and said, "Go ahead— flip your wig."

Laughter swept through the car as I made a big production of flipping that wig.

In the traffic jam next to us idled a truck full of

landscape workers. Well! When they saw this woman suddenly lose her hair, they all started laughing. I started laughing even harder, and everyone in our car joined in. It was such a liberating experience to know that people were laughing at me and I could join them in laughing at myself.

Trying to Make a Comeback

By the time I had been home for a month, I thought my roller-coaster ride was coming to an end. But the doctors insisted that it wasn't over yet. More radiation to my sternum area, requiring three weeks of treatment, needed to be done. Unfortunately, no hospital close to my home had the necessary radiation machine that regulated the depth of the rays' penetration into my skin. The closest facility was an hour's drive from my home.

I dreaded the daily drive to these treatments. My strength was only beginning to return. Driving that far took more energy than I had. So I enlisted the help of some friends and ladies of the church to drive me the first week. After that, my independence demanded that I drive myself.

Going back alone to the place where I had already been through so much trauma did not appeal to me. *How can I make the best of this?* I wondered. I picked up the phone. With my calendar in front of me, I called various doctors, nurses, and medical staff to make lunch appointments. The potentially morbid experience became something pleasant instead.

Dealing with My Fears

In returning to the hospital for my radiation treatment, my main fear was my tormenting thoughts. *What if the transplant didn't work?* How futile it would seem to have gone through such a radical procedure after so many other radical procedures and not have it work. How devastating that would be! *Maybe I should have left everything alone.*

I had soaring moments of trusting in the Lord and also crashing feelings of doubt and despair. I didn't know if this wild vacillation was exacerbated by the drastic metabolic chemical changes in my body and the resulting menopause, or if they were normal feelings of someone dealing with this disease.

Even though I believed very strongly in the Lord and I knew how he had preserved me through the ordeal, my faith didn't stop my mind from producing many haunting questions about death. *Maybe this is all there is. You live your human life for however long it is, and then you die, and you just go back to dust, and that's it.*

Sometimes I would sit outside in the night and be overcome with these morbid thoughts. I saw them as futile, painful, and sorrowful. It was as if I was testing my own faith in eternal life and the Word of God. Oh, how I struggled with my mortality. For quite a while I was convinced that death was the end of me, with no life thereafter. Perhaps I had been tasting death for so long that these sensations lingered.

But when I was really contemplative, when I would go all the way to the deepest part of my soul, I had this deep sense of belief. I believed in the resurrection of Jesus Christ and in the Word of God. I trusted that believers will be raised from the dead and go to be with the Lord. We all will be raised up to be like Jesus. Even though my sense of morbidity, mortality, and finality seemed so strong, what would ultimately win in my quest for truth was my strong conviction in the Word of God and the reality of the Resurrection.

Walks and Talks with My Neighbor

Some of the most important times during my healing were really the most simple things that a friend or neighbor would do for me. My neighbor Carol was one of those people. It was especially wonderful to have someone in my neighborhood to be this type of support for me, one who was there for me no matter what condition I was in physically or emotionally.

During all my ins and outs from the hospital or being home sick after treatment and surgery, she was always there—willing to help our family. Her faith, love, and kindness blessed our lives on a daily basis. For example, we used to be in a car pool together, and when I had to pull out of the car pool, Carol covered for me many times. She would drive the children and often kept them at her house after school. She provided for the need, whatever it was.

Because of her compassion and the fact that she also is raising three sons, I felt I could open up and talk with Carol about anything. Her eyes would well up with tears when I told her of my struggles—trying to raise three children, trying to recover myself as a normal person, and trying to live beyond the fear of recurrence of the disease. Carol spent many hours walking and talking with me. Her friendship helped my recovery process immensely.

Going Out into Public

Leaving my house was an adventure in humility. My blue isolation mask and bald head drew attention everywhere I went. I wanted desperately to be a normal person, yet my appearance made me look anything but normal. People didn't help my quest to feel normal. Many stared without any attempt to hide their curiosity. Some ventured a step further in rudeness. "Are we that bad?" asked some, with voices cold as ice. Others questioned, "Is your sense of smell so strong that you have to wear a mask?" or "Is the earth that bad that you have to isolate yourself?"

After a while, I responded to these inane comments with a blunt statement: "I'm wearing this because I'm suffering from radical treatment for cancer." When they heard this, they were startled and abashed. I hoped the next time they would be a little more gracious to those who are ill.

On the other hand, I could easily accept the inquisitiveness and stares from children. Their sense of curiosity had a sense of innocence and came from a natural desire to understand the complex world around them. For example, when I was in the grocery store, many children would ask, "Are you a doctor? Are you a nurse?" Or they would inquire, "Are you sick?" Or they would simply ask, "Why are you wearing that blue mask?" Their questions were graciously answered.

I most appreciated those people who let me be part of the crowd as they were. Those who let me pass by as if I had all my hair and no mask. On occasion, an interested person would ask a kind question, with an apology for intruding or possibly embarrassing me.

Often, as I walked from place to place, I continually and silently asked the Lord to give me long-suffering. I needed all I could get, for I was so tired of looking like a "geek"—the weird one in the crowd.

When my hair had grown to about one inch in length, I decided not to wear my wig and scarf anymore. I just puffed up my hair a little bit. At that time there was a popular rock star named Sinéad O'Connor, whom all the teenagers thought was so cool. During that summer girls were getting their hair cut real short to look like her.

Sometimes young people would tell me, "Oh, cool, you got your hair cut like Sinéad O'Connor!"

I'd say, "Well, not really, but I guess it's a look I can live with." I was happy someone famous had a hairstyle like mine. It helped me not feel like a woman with a butch haircut.

One day as I played tennis with my husband at our sports club, I wore my tennis dress but not my wig. A man who worked at the club later told me, "The first time I saw you out there playing a hard game of tennis with a bald head, I thought you were the neatest lady I ever saw in my life."

Another man who belonged to the same club suffered from premature balding. By the time he was twenty-three years old, he was totally bald. His baldness disturbed him, and he was very self-conscious about it. But when he met me and saw me running around with a little "fur" on my head and not being very self-conscious about it, it really liberated him. "If a woman can get through this," he said, "being bold and not caring what people think, surely I, as a man, can get through this."

Sometimes inspiring others, such as these men, helped me keep my head up and face life with a little more dignity.

Celebrating Survival

In July we had a lovely vacation at Cape Cod with Philip's family. Philip's brother, Rich, generously sent airfare for the five of us to fly to Boston so we could attend a family reunion. It was a special time to be united with Philip's grandmother, parents, brothers, and their families.

Philip's grandmother, Dorothy, had turned eighty-nine that year. So we offered a tribute to her and her longevity, honoring her as the matriarch of a wonderful family. We thanked God for her health and that she could be with the family at the Cape. My sister-in-law, Robin, gave a tribute and thanksgiving for my recovery. My father-in-law, Richard, called me a "miracle of God." Philip's cousin Trey and his wife, Nancy, were there from California with their adorable little daughter, Laura, who is a survivor of serious heart problems she endured as a little baby. There were five survivors there including Robin, a survivor of lupus, and my mother-in-law, also named Dorothy, who is blind in one eye.

It seemed this was a reunion of a special family, one that had every reason to celebrate survival and to celebrate life!

Helping a Woman Beat Cancer

My activities were very limited at the Cape. I couldn't run to the beach with everyone, nor could I join all their activities. But I didn't really mind. I enjoyed just being around the family as much as possible.

One day, while everybody was at the beach, I lounged in the shade by a pool. A woman named Joyce watched me move my chair into the shade every time the sun shifted. She finally came over to me and said, "I'm sorry to be so nosy, but I couldn't help noticing that here we are with our bathing suits on and you're trying to stay in the shade." She hesitated a moment, then added, "And you don't seem to have much hair."

"Yes," I replied, "I'm recovering from radical treatment for breast cancer."

I could tell she wanted to ask more questions about it, and I felt very comfortable talking with her because she was neither rude nor intrusive. Joyce told me how she had found a lump in her breast but intended on waiting to have it checked by a doctor.

"Don't wait," I told her. "Don't put it off. As soon as you get back home, make sure a doctor checks it out."

I heard from her after she had a biopsy done, and it turned out she did have breast cancer. When she called me, she was understandably upset. Her surgeon had advised her to have a mastectomy. I replied, "Whatever the doctor advises, do it." Then I urged, "Take the most aggressive treatment strategy they offer."

Fortunately, the cancer had not gone to her lymph nodes. Nevertheless, her surgeon and her oncologist put her on chemotherapy just to be safe. Joyce was extremely grateful that she had met me. My truthfulness had scared her into doing the right thing.

My Return to Piano Teaching

Due to the length of time involved in having a bone-marrow transplant, I had placed most of my piano students with other teachers. Their absence brought great sadness and emptiness into my life. Quite a few of my students had been with me four or five years. I had the joy of seeing them develop and become fine musicians, and we had become very close. My teaching methods included giving my students not only instruction in piano, but also my heart. So it was difficult not only for me to give up my students, but also for my students to give me up.

After the summer I felt strong enough to take back a few of my students. I called some of the families to find out if their children wanted to come back for piano lessons. A few students had refused to go to any other teacher, preferring to wait for my return. Some of these little children had insisted that I would get better and would be their piano teacher again. They told their parents, "We know that Mrs. Comfort is going to come back. God is going to bring Mrs. Comfort back to us." They had faith like strong lions. Parents told me how the children had prayed for me in their Sunday-school groups and had put my name in the prayer meetings at their church. Those who were Catholics had mentioned my name in the Mass for special prayers for healing.

This small group of ten students provided the opportunity for me to revive my piano studio in September. I knew I had to start out gradually. But I also knew these children came to me with a strong desire to learn and excel. I didn't have to push them along and thereby drain myself. All I had to do was teach; they, out of their own discipline and joy of learning, excelled week by week.

Teaching these children brought me such joy that I determined to be a piano teacher in spite of the fact that the radiation treatment had reduced the dexterity in my left hand. The resulting neuropathy (nerve damage), causing weakness in my left arm and hand, has been difficult to deal with after having practiced for so many years. I have kept myself away from the repertoire I used to play so that I wouldn't get too depressed—all the while hoping I would regain the function of my left hand and small motor skills so as to be dexterous enough to play the way I did before. I still have tingling sensations, discomfort, and impaired function of my left arm and hand, but I practice my piano and do the best I can with my limitation.

C h a p t e r

16

Determined to Live

As my recovery continued, a small thread of fear wove itself through every hour of every day. Multiplying cancer cells cannot be seen just by looking at a person, nor do they necessarily cause symptoms that the person would feel. Yet not seeing and not feeling do not mean that the cancer cells are not multiplying. My fear grew as I faced the six-month checkup following my bone-marrow transplant. I went through an arduous day of blood tests, X rays, and scans. Then I went home and nervously waited for the doctor's phone call.

"Well, Georgia," her familiar voice lilted over the phone, "it appears you are in remission. All the tests show the disease has not spread." She paused for a moment, then added, "Congratulations!"

My heart soared. I was so relieved that the disease had not taken any more toll on me. The doctor further informed me that my blood count and my whole general system seemed to be in very good shape in spite of the beating I had put it through.

Speaking to Medical Students

At the end of September my favorite doctor, the surgical oncologist, asked me to give a talk to the medical students at the medical center where I had undergone my bone-marrow transplant. He thought it would be good for the students to see patients as real, flesh-and-blood people who have lives outside of the hospital—lives away from dealing with cancer treatment. To complete this picture, he asked me also to play the piano. Wanting to give a decent performance, I selected two pieces—one by Chopin and another by Debussy—which required less left-hand facility.

When I asked how to prepare for the talk, the doctor said it would be a question-and-answer forum. "You don't have to prepare anything because they are just going to ask you questions. You only have to answer their questions."

On the day of the forum, I was introduced to the pathologist to whose class I had come to speak. After our greeting he said, "You have an hour-and-a-half to lecture."

I was stunned! "Lecture? I don't have any three-by-five cards or anything!" Before total panic set in, I remembered the Bible verse that tells us not to worry about what we are going to say because the Holy Spirit will give us the words to speak.

As I walked down the corridor I said, "Lord, I can't believe I'm going into a lecture hall filled with medical students, and I'm the one who is supposed to do the talking. Please, Lord, I open myself to You. I ask You to give me the words even at the last second, words that will benefit the students to make them learn, and words that can glorify You. Lord, please have the glory through this lecture."

Before I knew it—after that desperate little prayer—I was standing in front of a lecture hall full of students. Every pair of eyes stared expectantly. Someone handed me the microphone, and I began to speak.

I started by giving a chronological description of what had happened to me: before my diagnosis, at my diagnosis, and from then on. They interjected questions here and there, most of which dealt with psychological and spiritual concerns. Those questions afforded the Lord and me an opportunity to be able to share with them much more than the actual medical experiences I went through. I opened my heart and my spirit to give them a glimpse of how I emotionally survived all that I did. I told them I was a Christian, and I spoke about the power of God and the Spirit of the Lord.

One student asked me, "How have you been able to deal with the question, Why do bad things happen to good people?"

I told him, "I know there is a book with that title written by a Jewish rabbi concerning his child who died of a disease. I don't know how he resolved the problem. As for me, I really struggled with this question before I came to my own resolution." Then I told this student how my helicopter ride in Hawaii powerfully answered that question, how it changed my outlook and increased my desire to fight for life.

I finished my answer by sharing my motto with them—a verse from the Bible: "They that wait upon the Lord shall renew their strength. They shall mount up with wings like eagles; they shall run and not be weary; they shall walk and not faint" (Isaiah 40:31). I was ready to fly.

At the end of the lecture I said, "There are three people I would really like to honor. Number one, I would like to honor God. The reason I would like to honor God is that He is my Maker and He is your Maker."

"Furthermore," I said, "it's during times like the one I went through that you can really get to know how real our great God is. Without His power I would not have been able to survive. This life is more than what we know. Being a human being here on earth is part of an eternal plan. Life goes on and is much more than we can even fathom. So I want to honor God for who He is and for all He has been to me. He is eternal, and He is powerful."

"Next," I continued, "I would like to honor my husband, Philip, who has shown me unconditional love through this whole ordeal. When I looked so terrible after the bone-marrow transplant, he would hold me and tell me that I was his beautiful girl. I want to honor my husband for such unconditional love."

"Finally," I said, "I want to honor my oncology surgeon for being not only an excellent surgeon but also someone who was willing to guide me and care for me. He was my friend, especially during my severe crisis."

After I finished speaking, the students gathered around me. Many of them were crying. Throughout their undergraduate and medical training, they had never heard a woman telling them that she was not just a miracle of modern medicine but a miracle of God. The reality of God touched their spirits.

I left the remarkable event emotionally uplifted and physically fatigued. I knew it had been worth it to have touched many medical students' lives by sharing with them the reality of the Lord's power and purpose. A week later I received a beautiful flower arrangement from these medical students, with a large homemade card filled with personal notes of thanksgiving.

Chapter

Overcoming Despair

In the dark, alone times of the bone-marrow transplant unit, I had made a promise to God. As I stared at the bare ceiling or at the posters and cards on my wall, I vowed never to forget those women who would have to suffer the same pain, loneliness, fear, and indignity.

During October and November, six months after my transplant, I began to receive calls from patients who were considering a bone-marrow transplant as treatment for their cancer. My doctors had begun to refer their patients to me, believing I could provide hope and inspiration to them in their fight against cancer.

I gave my attention to these women, despite the fatigue I experienced by continually relating my story and empathizing with them. I considered the opportunity a blessing. I understood their fears, and I wanted to be there for them. I remembered too well my own unsuccessful search for women who had survived a bone-marrow transplant. I wanted to be that surviving role model for others.

I spoke to many of these women. I helped calm the fears of women terribly frightened by what would lie ahead. I shared the gospel of Jesus Christ with some and listened to all. Three of these women died, making me even more thankful that I had spent time with them.

Of all the women I have seen battle cancer, Christians fare the best. They endure the treatment with a better attitude and a certain buoyancy. Cancer is a huge giant, an attacking monster. Nothing seems bigger than cancer growing in one's body. Only the healing power of Christ—the same power that raised Him from the dead—can beat it. People who don't have the knowledge of the Lord Jesus Christ in their lives feel helpless and powerless. These feelings of helplessness and powerlessness seem to allow the disease to take over rapidly.

Of course, not all who believe in Jesus Christ will be healed physically. But my observation is that those who are believers have a better attitude and sense of well-being than those who do not. I believe that these attributes can really make a difference, giving more time and possibly allowing the disease to be overcome and cured. I have seen it and heard it in the lives of other people and in my own life. It really does make a big difference. Those people who know the Lord do much better in dealing with the disease than those who don't.

That's why I beseech everyone who is struggling with a terminal disease to receive the gospel of Jesus Christ. Without the knowledge of the saving power of Christ and assurance of eternal life with Him, people are in a desperate situation. I have seen women rapidly taken over by the disease when their spirit was down and their sense of hope was gone. And I have seen women recover when their spirit was vivified by hope in Christ.

My friend Becky had breast cancer and, unfortunately, her disease started to spread. She eventually decided to undergo a bone-marrow transplant. In her battle, she nearly died of a fungal pneumonia. Her situation was medically hopeless, but she did not lose her hope in the Lord! She miraculously recovered. In fact, she has made medical history! I, with so many others, prayed for her, and the Lord heard our prayers. She is a living testimony of Christ's risen life, as I am.

Remember, *probabilities* can be depressing and keep us from achieving wellness, but *possibilities* can give us inspiration, hope, joy, and a fighting spirit! May we *live!* And may we find strength in the power of God.

A High Risk for Recurrence?

By giving myself to these women I experienced joy—but also exhaustion and increased anxiety. In fact, the most unfortunate result of becoming a part of their lives was that I became involved with many women who were dying of cancer and who did not have successful transplants. This continual contact with cancer and painful memories augmented my own anxiety and fear about recurrence.

It usually takes a year to know whether or not the transplant was successful—and even five years to know whether or not there was a cure. This knowledge, coupled with the ill women I counseled, made it impossible to silence the nagging fear that haunted my thoughts: *What if my treatment didn't work?*

One of my doctors had been watching how I coped with the disease. One day he asked, "Georgia, since you have such a high risk for recurrence, how can you be so happy?"

Inside, I felt he had slugged me. *"High risk for recurrence?"* I tried not to think about that. *I went through all this so I wouldn't be high risk for recurrence. How can you equate my happiness with that?* I thought. I let my response to his question come out slowly, "I'm happy because I want to be happy with the days I have left."

Since I really didn't know how many days I had left, I felt this manic energy racing through me. I wanted to live as much as I could, so I adopted this premise: "I've got to do all the living I can now—especially since I'm feeling good and I have some energy." I wanted to go for the gusto and live it up, even though I still had to wear my mask in public. I joined a tennis league and went to dance classes again. I became involved in all the boys' sports activities. I wanted to be involved in my church and play the piano again in church meetings. I rehabilitated myself as best I could as a pianist, and I was determined to be a good piano teacher.

During November all the energy I expended left me with little resistance to infection. I developed a sinus infection that turned into an upper respiratory bronchial infection. Radiation had so damaged my bronchi on the left that, once I developed a bad infection in that area, it took a long time to heal.

Brenda's Death

As the November days grew shorter, eight months after my transplant, darkness seeped into my soul. While my exhausted physical body fought the bronchial infection, my spirit fought the darkness of yet another emotional battle when Brenda, a friend from my church, died of ovarian cancer.

When Brenda had been diagnosed with ovarian cancer at the age of thirty-two, her disease was very advanced. Amazingly and miraculously, she lived for two years beyond her prognosis. Brenda went through hell. She was constantly on chemotherapy. She was the only person I ever met who had chemotherapy and didn't lose her hair. Brenda had beautiful, long brown hair. Knowing she was needed by her husband and children, she maintained a strong sense of dignity throughout her ordeal. Near the end, her frail, tiny body had such a huge, distended abdomen you would have thought she was ten months pregnant.

To the very end, until she had to be hospitalized, she tried to live a normal life. She went to work, set her hair, and always looked good. She tried her very best to be involved with her children's activities. She was an incredible woman. She had such a heart for people that she opened her home in hospitality to many, caring for others while she suffered. She was a real testimony of expressing grace in the midst of suffering and a testimony of Christian perseverance.

I loved Brenda dearly. We had become very close as we walked this path together, suffering with each other and trying to encourage each other. One morning when I went to visit Brenda in the hospital, she was sitting in a chair by the window. Her eyes were shining; her face was gaunt yet joyful. She was happy to share with me that she had seen a beautiful vision in the clouds that morning. She felt that she had been given a glimpse into eternity through the clouds, and she felt very hopeful about life after death. While her grief was the thought of leaving her family, her joy was the thought of living eternally with Christ in glory.

Brenda had taken a turn for the worse in October, dying a few weeks later. Her death deeply affected me. I grieved because I had lost another dear friend and because she had to leave behind a wonderful husband and two beautiful children. I also feared that I might be the next to go. There had been three of us. Barbara went, Brenda went—and I felt like I was at the deli with number 3 in my hand. How could I be so presumptuous as to think that I was going to beat this disease?

My belief that I had been healed began to weaken. I became very depressed, thinking, *Why fight? It's a terrible disease. It's a killer disease. Look what happened to my friends. How can I escape?*

Brenda's Funeral

Prior to Brenda's funeral I told the women from our church, "I hope you aren't offended if I don't go to the funeral, but I just don't think I can handle it. My emotions are so drained."

The grim reality of how this horrible disease kills so many young women overwhelmed me. I thought of the other women who were fighting for their lives—it was all so sad. I grieved deeply for all of us.

I planned not to go to Brenda's funeral. But a few hours before the funeral I was thinking of Brenda—

how much I loved her and what a wonderful Christian sister she had been to me. I could not justify skipping her funeral, even though I had so many good reasons to not go. So I went.

I sobbed and sobbed from the minute I stepped into the church, releasing my pent-up emotions. And then I realized that I was lamenting not only Brenda's death but also Barbara's. I had never fully grieved Barbara's death because I was in the hospital at the time. During the phase after the bone-marrow transplant when I had heard about Barbara's death, I had stifled my emotions because my strength was so fragile. Allowing the tears to flow heavily at that time would have been really bad for the healing process. So I had shut down my emotions, putting them on hold, because I didn't think my body could handle it. Now at Brenda's funeral I grieved deeply for both of my friends, finally able to cry out all my deepest feelings for the loss of both of them.

When I walked by Brenda's open casket, I honored Barbara too. I congratulated both of them. It seems to me that dying is probably the most difficult thing a person can do. So I congratulated them that they had suffered, died, and made it through. I had a deep realization that both of them were with the Lord. I wasn't sure if they had met each other in heaven, yet I wouldn't be surprised.

One of the ministers who spoke at Brenda's funeral said, "Brenda is like a ship who is now on the other shore. At one time, this ship was on our shore, and we could see her. Her departure doesn't mean there is no more Brenda; it means that the ship has gone beyond the horizon and is no longer in our sight."

These words comforted me. I then realized that Brenda and Barbara and all the other Christian women I have known who have died are on another shore—yet they still *are*. They have a different kind of existence, and we don't know what it is like. But we do know that they are with Jesus on another shore. With this realization I left the funeral uplifted.

But those thoughts didn't completely put an end to my darkness and grieving. For three weeks I continued mourning. I found that I also grieved for myself—for what I had been through. While taking the treatment, I had tried so hard to be positive and to be cheerful for my family. I had never allowed myself to sink all the way down into the massive pool of emotional pain. But now in the recovery period, I often would hide my grief, then go to my room to weep in agony.

In December I reached bottom. I continued to be sick, and my emotions floundered in the darkness. I was very confused, depressed, and grieving. I found it difficult to get out of this state of being.

Trying to Find a Way Out

The one thing I looked forward to was our family reunion at Christmas. I hoped this holiday could help get me out of my depression. My mother, sister, and I decided that the reunion should be held on an island off the Gulf coast of Mexico.

Everyone on my side of the family—my husband

and sons, my parents, my sister Sally and her son, Ben, and my two brothers, Bob and Ted—met in this tropical paradise for the Christmas holidays. The island was a paradise, but our vacation was a disaster for the adults. My sister and parents got very sick. I came home with a worse bronchial infection than when I had left. At least my sons and their cousin Ben had a good time!

My hometown greeted us with subzero conditions. I didn't know how I was going to make it. I seemed to be in a physical and emotional abyss.

On my fortieth birthday, January 8, 1991, a longtime friend of mine, Kathy, called me from her home in Albuquerque, New Mexico. She had heard that I was sick, and she offered me a round-trip ticket to Albuquerque and a luxurious condominium all to myself. What a great present sent from heaven—it was just what I needed!

I arrived late at night, so I didn't open the drapes in my bedroom until morning. Kathy had told me that the condo was near the mountains, but I didn't think about that when I arrived. But the next morning, when I opened the drapes, I was elated at the spectacular view of the mountains! I immediately thought that this must be what it will be like when we pass from this life to the next. Presently we are veiled, but one day the veil will be lifted. We will see with incredible awe the reality of the life to come.

While in Albuquerque, although I spent some time with Kathy and her family, I had many hours to myself. I used the time to take care of myself, to rest, to take walks, and to pray. During some prayer sessions, I had some extraordinary spiritual experiences. I was desperate to get out of the deep emotional, psychological, and physical pit I had tumbled into. Nothing but prayer seemed to lift me out.

One night I prayed intently for our soldiers in the Persian Gulf; the war had just broken out. I begged the Lord to preserve the soldiers and exercise His sovereignty over the war. Then I wanted to pray for myself, but I didn't know what to say. So I opened myself to allow the Holy Spirit to pray for me. The prayer must have gone on for an hour, without me knowing exactly what was prayed through me. I felt the Spirit flow through my being with a mighty rush. I felt extremely energized. I uttered words in a different language, seemingly transported to a different place. After that I felt strengthened, refreshed, renewed, and even healed in a new kind of a way. I couldn't pinpoint exactly what had been healed, but I sensed that I had received more of a healing. And I sensed that the Spirit had prayed through me that night.

Thanks to the gift from my friends Kathy and Gary and to the uplifting power of prayer, I left Albuquerque feeling physically and spiritually ready to face the challenges ahead.

I Believe the True Report

After I started to recover from the chronic bronchitis, I again began to reach out to some of the women I had met through my doctors' referrals. Many of these women were trying to decide whether or not to do a bone-marrow transplant as a treatment for breast cancer. They were all dear, wonderful women, most of them in their late thirties or early forties. Being in a crisis situation, they were willing to do anything to save their lives.

I developed relationships with many of them through writing letters of encouragement, calling them, and allowing them to call me to talk about what they were going through. I frequently had the opportunity to share the gospel with them. I spoke to them about death, the afterlife, and eternal life. Some of these women were Christians who needed their faith renewed and strengthened. Those who weren't Christians heard the gospel.

During this time, some of these women were dealing with the fact that their bone-marrow transplant had not been completely successful. Some of these women had to receive more chemotherapy right after their transplant because some cancer remained in their system. What a heartache! They had suffered so much already, and now they had to suffer more.

In March I was due for my one-year checkup after the bone-marrow transplant. At that time I would find out how effective the transplant had been for me. If the women I had befriended had received more positive reports, I would have been less anxious. But I never forgot that, when I went in for my bone-marrow transplant, I had found no positive role models to encourage me. And I still didn't have that positive role model. As a result, by the time of my one-year checkup, my anxiety had grown to enormous proportions. I tried to be trusting and restful, to act as if nothing were bothering me, but I was full of anxiety and overcome with anguish.

One evening shortly before the tests, I was with Philip in our living room. The tension snapped. I blurted out, "Philip, I don't want to die. Oh Philip, what if my reports aren't good? How will I handle it? I don't want to die, Philip." As we cried together, we realized that there was nothing we could do about it. It was going to be the way it was. Whether the report was good or not good, we just had to accept it.

During my years of illness, I had discovered that when I am in a crisis situation and my fears are swelling and my anxiety is high, it helps to cry and then pray. One of my favorite prayers has been: "God, grant me the courage to change the things I can, the serenity to accept the things I cannot change, and the wisdom to know the difference." Many times when I wanted to take control and change something, I would remember this prayer, hoping that the Lord would give me the wisdom to know what I really could change and what I couldn't—and the grace to accept what I couldn't.

My One-Year Checkup

I went to the hospital for my checkup. The tests were comprised of a bone scan, a chest scan, a lower abdomen scan, and a chest X ray. I could still feel the anxiety swirling around inside me. As I was driving home and coming around a curve on the freeway, I remember asking the Lord to give me the grace to accept whatever the news was going to be. I then had an overwhelming sense that the scan results would be good and that I needed to hold on to the initial belief, "With His stripes I am healed." I needed to hold on to the reality of what the Lord had done in my life. All the experiences of the other women and all my own fears about the results had obfuscated the reality of what the Lord had done for me. All the dark clouds of doubt and depression had obscured my view.

As I came around the bend I sensed those dark clouds of fear and depression lifting from me. I started sobbing and claimed again all the promises in the Bible that I had been claiming for the past year. As I looked up toward heaven, the beautiful clouds in the sky appeared to be light and bright. I started praising the Lord and thanking Him for saving me and healing me. I exclaimed, "Lord, I want to believe in You. I don't want to believe in any report." I started to sing the song "I Believe the True Report."

As I sang this song, I realized that the true report was my faith in Christ. My true report about my physical condition was: I am healed. The Lord had done a marvelous work in my life. I had superimposed the other women's relapses onto my own life. In so doing, I had been tricked by the enemy into thinking I was doomed. I cried out, "Lord, forgive me for living according to what I see and for not living according to faith in Your Word and what You think."

All the way home I felt great relief and peace. I said, "Lord, no matter what my doctors say, I want to believe You. I want to believe this true report."

Good News

"Every test result is clear," my medical oncologist said on the phone about seven o'clock that same evening. I was so happy I could hardly believe it! Even though I had such a wonderful time riding home believing and praising the Lord, another part of me held back from accepting this report. It was so hard for me to believe that I could be one of the rare ones—that out of so many women who had metastatic breast cancer, I was free of disease. I thought it strange that I had gotten the results so quickly, and I wondered if the doctor had looked at my scans thoroughly. Sensing my anxiety, she also told me that I needed to see a psychologist.

Even those thoughts didn't stop the flow of emotion. I sobbed and sobbed tears of relief. And then I joined my family in their excitement. That evening Philip, the boys, and I stood around the dining-room table holding hands. We all cried for joy, lifting our hands up and praising the Lord. One by one each person thanked the Lord and gave Him the glory. It was a wonderful, joyous time. It seemed like a thousand pounds had been lifted off of the family, and the clouds of darkness and fear and anxiety that had been settling in were dispelled.

Realizing It Was True

Even though I received the good report I had prayed for, the reality did not immediately sink in. It took me two or three days of continually speaking the Word of God—and continually claiming that I did believe in what the Lord had done in my life—before I fully accepted the good news. I suppose this was because I had been startled by hearing the news so quickly—it usually takes two or three days—and because I had grown accustomed to bad news in the past. It was too good to be true. But, finally, my whole heart and soul started realizing that—*yes!*—what I claimed and believed had actually happened. There was no evidence of cancer in my body!

Isn't that amazing! We can suffer such radical treatment and eventually feel good. I feel very good now, two years after my transplant. My yearly checkup indicates that I am in remission. There is no sign of cancer anywhere in my body! The area in my sternum that had been damaged by cancer is completely restored. I am a miracle of modern medicine and the power of God! What good news!

to Georgia:

the Greeks like moderns
celebrated the games
and sang of them in panegyric praise—
the winners were heroes
eulogized in Olympic odes
immortalized above the gods—
the marathoner was the best of them
if he could outlast the rest and win.
the wreath he earned would never fade
because its garland was laud and praise.

but what of those unsung
who were forced to run a marathon
or fight for life in a wild arena
and battle invisible odds?
what crown is given to them
for wrestling thoughts and slaying giants
for testing limits and trying time?

if they fall we drop a petal on their grave
and grieve the failure as our own.
but if they rise they flower praise
and wear the victor's living wreath
a laureate of grace and peace
for those triumphant, tired, and meek!

march 18, 1991

The National Cancer Society sponsors a program
called Look Good, Feel Better. Throughout the year

following my transplant, a representative from the society visited me. Each time, she took photographs of me to show my process of getting back to my life, becoming active again, and doing things I did before. She also helped me take care of my physical appearance after my chemotherapy treatments. Her whole concept is, if you try to make yourself look good, you will feel better.

Later the representative planned to show the photographs as a slide presentation for 350 women at a formal luncheon. She asked me if I would be there to give a little talk at the end. It was good timing, because just a few days before I had received the news that there was no evidence of the disease in my body.

I started out my talk by emphasizing to the women the importance of early detection of breast cancer. The women who have the best survival rate are those who are fortunate enough to have the cancer detected early. With a lumpectomy or mastectomy, they can often live for years and be fine. I told them not to neglect getting regular mammograms and, if they were to find a lump, to take it seriously.

I went on to talk about how grateful I was to have received the best of modern medicine and God's wonderful power. I told them that I was a miracle of medicine and a miracle of God. As I spoke, I received more confirmation from the Spirit of what the Lord had actually done in my life. At that moment I was enlivened with the desire to testify to the wonderful power of the resurrected Christ. As I spoke about my present wellness, I couldn't help but give the glory to God.

When I finished speaking, the women rose to their feet and began to applaud. When everyone was on their feet, I couldn't say another word. I stood there weeping, immersed in the Holy Spirit and bathed in the love of God. I felt the Lord had received the glory, and the women had received encouragement to seek the best modern treatment available for breast cancer and to depend upon the power of God. That experience confirmed what the Lord had done in my life.

For right now, I have won the battle. I have fought desperately to gain a few more good years, and I plan to appreciate and celebrate every minute God gives me on this earth. But someday my time will come, and my soul will go home. I don't need to worry that my soul will get lost. Just as a monarch butterfly makes a solo flight for thousands of miles to its exact destination, where it meets with myriads of other monarchs that also made the flight . . . and just as the tiny bone-marrow cells knew how to go home . . . so will my soul. When it is my time, I will go to the other shore where Barbara, Brenda, and Ryan—and Jesus— have gone ahead.

Georgia Comfort's experiences are documented in a brief video presentation entitled *Bone-Marrow Transplant: A Fighting Chance.* Her description of the physical and emotional stress encountered during the procedure will benefit any cancer patient contemplating or about to undergo a bone-marrow transplant. In addition to a positive mental attitude, Georgia stresses the importance of a strong spiritual faith during treatment. Support from medical professionals, family, and friends, as well as pleasant, comfortable surroundings are also significant factors for recovery. The nine-minute video is available from:

Health Sciences Consortium
201 Silver Cedar Court
Chapel Hill, NC 27514
(919) 942-8731